I0505725

Micronutrient Happiness

Increase Your Nutrient Density & Crack the Code for Joy!

Barbara Christensen

The time is now to seek your happiness.

Copyright © 2019 by Barbara Christensen.

All rights reserved. No part of this publication may be reproduced, distributed or transmitted in any form or by any means, including photocopying, re-cording, or other electronic or mechanical methods, without the prior written permission of the publisher, except in the case of brief quotations embodied in critical reviews and certain other noncommercial uses permitted by copy-right law. For permission requests, write to the publisher, addressed "Attention: Permissions Coordinator," at the web address below.

Barbara Christensen
www.PaleoVegeo.com

Book Layout ©2019 BookDesignTemplates.com

Disclaimer:
Barbara Christensen, the sole creator of 'Micronutrient Happiness", is not a medical doctor. The author is not engaged in rendering professional advice or services to the individual reader. This book is for entertainment purpose only.

The ideas, procedures, and suggestions contained within this work are not intended as a substitute for consulting with your physician. All matters in regards to your health require medical supervision. The author shall not be liable or responsible for any loss or damage allegedly arising from any in-formation or suggestions within this book. You, as someone that has reached out to me as a life coach, are totally and completely responsible for your own health and healthcare. Take your health seriously and if you have medical issues talk to your doctor before starting this or any nutritional or physical program.

Micronutrient Happiness / Barbara Christensen.. —1st ed.. -- 1st ed.
ISBN 979-8-6014691-9-7

For those in my soul family, my testers in all things crazy and woo-woo. You allow me to take the sad stupidity of judgements, and change it into the energy of joy with total ease. I could never do any of this whole heartedly without you.
Love is always the answer.

Epigenetics doesn't change the genetic code, it changes how that's read. Perfectly normal genes can result in cancer or death. Vice-versa, in the right environment, mutant genes won't be expressed. Genes are equivalent to blueprints; epigenetics is the contractor. They change the assembly, the structure.

—BRUCE LIPTON

DISCLAIMER: Let me cover the bases before we get started. As a holistic   fitness & wellness professional with several decades of experience working with people to create change in their lives, I believe 100% in what I'm sharing within this book. I know that the clinical studies and research I'm sharing with you will open your mind to something different, and hopefully something that gives you some hope and possibilities that weren't there before today.

However, given that people are nowadays super-litigious and enjoy suing people for practically any reason they can I'm going to go through the boring legal blurb that, sadly, needs to be done to protect me from someone who says they got ill because they were asked to banish all of the toxic, chemically created, additive laced, denatured stuff that lines the supermarket shelves, use organically essential oils and encapsulated natural supplements, and instead to eat only fresh, natural and unaltered foods that come from non-toxic soil (organically created like they were), and if you aren't vegan, which swims in rivers or the sea wildly, walks on land eating pastures and bugs, or flies in the air.

I know it sounds utterly ridiculous (and it is) but there are people who will claim that removing known toxins, allergens and irritants from their food and from their bodies will, in some way have harmed them, caused mental anguish or removed the fundamental human right to freedom of choice.

Even more insane, some clever creatures will get a smart enough lawyer to press a case, win and repossess my home, my car and all my other stuff and stick me in jail for the rest of my natural life. (I'm only half joking!).

Therefore, read the following statement BEFORE you read the rest of this book or follow any of the advice given.

The elimination process and diet advice given within these pages is for information purposes only and in no way supersedes any prior advice given by a medical practitioner, registered dietician or nutritionist.

Should you follow the advice herein you are choosing to do so of your own free will, without coercion and in the full knowledge that the dietary or lifestyle recommendations in this book have not been personally designed for you and that should you suffer from a medical condition of any kind or suspect that the dietary regimen may cause you a medical problem of any kind that you should speak to a qualified medical practitioner for advice.

Further, if you choose to follow the dietary or lifestyle recommendations and feel that it is affecting you adversely or that you are feeling negative side effects in any way then you should cease it immediately and consult your doctor.

That's it! It's unfortunate that it's necessary but now you've been told.

The rest is up to you...

CONTENTS

Finding Happiness

So let's start with what this book was meant to address, happiness. Happiness feels so unknown to many of us, and it is because we don't really address the vision of loving ourselves without emotionally unraveling.

What is this idea of the unknown? What is your fear, shame, guilt, the dark emotions that are blocking the whispers in your life that are there to lead you into your happiness? They (the choices you let happen to you rather than choosing) all drip from fear.

Fear is the biggest lie that we have in our being, and yet even as a life coach I have lived a half-life filled with fear. I let these dark emotions lead me into every one of the hard decisions in my life, and walk away from everything that was just too scary to believe. I let fear lead me into my high school sweetheart's arms. I knew he wasn't the one for me, but I was fearful about what if I walked through high school without ever having a serious boyfriend. I also let that fear lead me into some situations with him that should have been red flags, but I was already there. Already in the coupling. Lesson of my childhood is that you never uncouple just to uncouple. There has to be a really really bad thing to walk you away from anyone that offers you love. My mom had told me over and over that she only divorced my dad because he felt so much guilt over the way he acted while she was pregnant with my sister, that he stopped paying any attention to my brothers and me. So his alcoholism, cheating, lying, refusing to work, physical and verbal abuse weren't enough to walk away. So with all of the knowing of my childhood I spent most of my senior year following the lost soul of a boyfriend around, begging for his love until I would finally get it. We live in the present even if we rewire through the past.

I also allowed fear to lead me into dropping the AP classes where I felt I didn't belong (and leaving the band). Had I stayed with those classes I could have easily gotten a scholarship into college. Instead I still have no degree. I have completed diploma course work, and have a Cosmetology license, but what an amazing N.D. I would have made! See it is easier to walk away than challenge yourself to belong within a group when you carry the dragging energy of your wounded soul. When you walk in the energy of not being enough, you walk with fear in your heart. So it wasn't just fear that I would fail those classes, it was a shame that I wasn't enough. Fear births shame. I have let fear lead me into the darkest spaces in my lifetime, and there it has clung to every cell in my being refusing to release its darkness, refusing to release my heart. It duplicated over and over again into shame, and that shame allowed me to be a shrinking violet and to make every decision to shrink down into a space where I couldn't be seen.

When fear grows, it lets shame bloom. I let shame lead me into giving up the most sacred beliefs that I had in this life. I let shame lead me into the drinking problem I had in high school, and they continued for many many years after that because alcohol is a numbing agent. Brené Brown says that shame is a focus of self. I think that it's the focus on all of the beliefs we have about our existence. Recently a friend of mine also said that shame is the feeling that we are a bad person and unlovable because we make mistakes. So unlovable and so many mistakes is what I felt in most of my life. This feeling of being unlovable was both emotionally saying to not love me first, but also bloomed because of what I was feeding and feeling in this body. When you get that deep into being unlovable then all that is left is to try to numb the pain. So alcohol, and bad micronutrients, and of course shame lead me into bad relationship after bad relationship with people, food and life choices.

These relationships weren't just about human interaction; it was food, career and any life decision that came along. Occasionally I would take the safer path because I needed to come up for air. Yet I still sought out what would verify that I was the great mistake within the universe. The twin flames don't stay so check mark on that verification. Finding the right fit I still walk away from it, so of course check mark on not being good enough. Eventually all of us will take all of that baggage into a longer holding relationship. Thankfully for me that wasn't with food, but with human relationships that I assumed would finally put an end to the shame. How many of you have walked your shame forward into a life without a thought about what you were really creating with those emotions? I am talking about any relationship in your life that is connected to your emotions.

What I didn't realize is that when you bring fear and shame into a relationship, it sparks a friend. That friend is guilt, and guilt gives you every opportunity to rise up and bring it along when you are living in that toxic emotional sludge. Guilt lets you continue to make mistakes to bring home the dream of being a mistake. To bring home the belief that you are truly not worthy of the highest power of love. Guilt lets you eat the box of donuts, and then feel so badly that you will eat another.

I have guilt for not being enough within my family unit. I have guilt for not being enough of a loving child. I have guilt for letting myself into situations where I allowed myself to be victimized. I have guilt for not being enough to be a real mother, and then not being enough when I finally became a mother. I have guilt for spending the first half of my life in rushed relationships trying to run from real love, and the second half of my life asleep. I think we can all admit that parenting is about rushing through life and sleeping through it, or wishing for it to speed by so we can finally sleep.

As humans we waste time, and I am no different than all of the rest of the humans out there. I have guilt for what I eat, and I have guilt for when I don't eat. I have guilt for wanting to be happy, and I have guilt for being sad. I have guilt for mentioning my truths, and guilt for wanting to hide them. I have so much guilt that I ended up living like a bad apology for far too long in life rather than living in the truth of what I truly desire. Every day starts to feel the same and you live in this grey world where your choices are incomplete, and also unknown.

This is the way that we create disease within our body and our soul. I want you to realize that all of these dark emotions get stuck within and they slowly become all that remain. When you are feeling so poorly within your machine body, and you can't figure it out, that unknown is all of this that I am sharing with you.

So what happens when you feel a spark in life?

When you are living in this bland, grey life and something shiny comes along, you don't want to believe it. How many times have you been in a moment of truth that this was your calling, this is your purpose, this will help me, this will heal me, this is the greatest possibility you have come across. You bring up first the guilt. If I am happy, how many mistakes will I have to make to create this? Then you bring in the shame. For me to choose for myself is the most selfish thing on the planet. I can't afford it, and I am not worth it. Then you bring up the fear. Most likely it isn't even meant for you. You aren't enough, you aren't enough, and you aren't enough. So you just pull all of that energy within, creating a deeper crater in your heart chakra, and walk back into the dark. This isn't a book that is going to delve much further into this psychological space beyond the connection to nutrients, but I wanted to address the fact that you are walking into this opportunity for change with a huge group of pre-defined reasons to keep being unhappy, and as the song says, "bury the sunlight". If you can't see the sunlight, then you leave it all unknown. Living in the unknown is going to seem easier, but in truth it isn't.

If you can look beyond this unknown, and finally start looking into your awareness, what is happiness?

I have asked myself that a lot over the last few years. I finally started to see the truth in it at the end of this last year. I realized that it isn't a number. I was just turning fifty and within twenty pounds of my highest weight. I created beliefs that this was all about metabolism, of course about being old, about not eating the right foods, and I fell into sadness. If a fifty year old certified personal trainer and nutritional therapist cannot be her healthiest being, then isn't it just a waste of time to keep trying?

I created this state of being. I sat one day and thought about that, without putting the fear, shame or guilt into it. I know what happens to me at the end of a year because as an empathic and intuitive individual, the holiday season is a beast for me to get through, anyway. Yet somehow in that moment of emotional trauma, I opened up a tiny awareness in my body and it started seeking truth.

This was an awakening, and that the truth about happiness really is about it being something I already had inside of me. It took me back to four years previously when I changed my supplements. For the first time in decades I felt almost no anxiety (except for the empathic part) and a sparked feeling of happiness. Just by giving into something that I had felt my body needed, I gave myself the love that it truly desired. That was a huge vibrational shift.

Everything is vibrations. Vibrations can bring us up, and they can wipe us out. My belief that I was suddenly unhappy, unwell, unattractive was not facts. It was, as any of you that have read "The Secret" can attest to, just a belief. I was buying into all of the low vibrational fruit and it was leading me into the darkness. I had walked up to a door, and allowed a deep soul connection to open me up to the truth. What was it that I had created in this body that I could now change?

Anything can be your spark of truth. At that point my spark was a smile and I started the process of asking for more. Universe, what am I seeking, can you show me? Universe, what does my body desire? Universe, what turns me on? Universe, what brings me joy? The universe started to answer in ways I never imagined. With just one smile I was reminded of who I am, and I started releasing the toxic sludge and opening up to what else was possible in this life.

This brought dance back into my life by way of Maxine Jones. She is an amazing lady I had never heard of from the UK. Then like a domino she brought Sally Bee into my life, which is a joy on a daily basis with the most positive attitude you could ever wish for. It brought me happy lights, sauna blankets, vibration plates, intermittent fasting. I started to do my hair again, and put on makeup. It brought me a surprise in the love of my own body, which I maybe have never truly had before. I started talking to my body, asking it what it wanted, and slowly over a year's time I released all of the information for this book ... and twenty pounds.

I am not ready for that to be the end of my story, so I am also smart enough to be getting all of the blood work, urine work, poop work done for my body. This book isn't about overlooking the tools in life that can help you dig deeper into what your body needs. This book is about going into the space to start creating an awareness of where you want to go in this life and what your body craves to create this joy. We can be everything, but not to everyone. We can be everything, but the truth is do you want to be? The biggest takeaway I have found is that creation takes energy and joy, and that you don't have to be everything. You just need to love yourself.

Creation, like rewiring your body, takes allowing **you** to be worth the work, and to let yourself be loved when you think you are unlovable. It is about letting go of the fear to go after the life that is calling you into happiness. I also remain strongly confident that highly vibrational plants are the simplest way to increase this vitality in your body, while you are working emotionally on the rest. I wanted to write this book about this area that so many of us find confusing... micronutrients, which will impact your happiness far quicker than just about anything else in life. This book is just the tip of that iceberg.

Macronutrients are the easy part. They are listed on everything and there are apps galore to use to guide you in determining which macro set is right for you. Macronutrients are fats, carbohydrates and proteins. When I created my Ketolicious Reset program two years ago I talked to my clients a lot about macronutrients, and how important getting enough carbohydrates truly is. Those healthy carbohydrates are what create a healthy microbiome.

The microbiome is the alien life force within that is responsible for your immune support, your neurotransmitters, and so much more. Yet as a nation we are dumping them into the sea and relying on saturated fats, those animal and manufactured fats that we have determined will create the weight loss we desire.

What a no-carb diet will do to a person that doesn't need to follow it for a medical reason, is dump out all of the toxins from your cells - and they will find other homes. I believe we are doing to see a rise in deadly diseases that are going to be linked to this toxic rush out of our cells without the functional micronutrients that the body needs to metabolize and release them. Skinny sludge is not what I desire for you. Healthy and happy is what will give you the best quality of life, and hopefully a long life at that. I am not saying that there isn't a benefit in lowering your high carbohydrate existence, or that our brains don't enjoy fats. However, we do need to support our functional bodies, and we are not really all sure how to do that.

Carbs are the fiber that will pull toxins through the intestinal tract, fermenting and feeding your good bacteria, and clear out your colon on the way out. Food is the common denominator for us all. We all have to eat. We all live in these soft, sensual bodies that overall work the same for each of use. Yes, we have some mutations that make us different, some ancestry that will make you different from me. That is where the macronutrient really should come into play. However the antioxidants, vitamins, minerals and synergies that we haven't even discovered in whole foods; these are what will create the magic within you.

You are of the universe. Like the stars, and trees, the soil and the air we breathe ... you are made up of something quite unique. This Mother Earth has provided everything we, as bodies, need to be. So now is the time to return to the micronutrient foundation that will give you the happiness and awareness to give back to the Earth before we are not able to turn things around.

In this book I am going to take you through some of my personal experiences, as well as give you the science that I can show points to how nutrition is essential for this elevated consciousness and what it does for our body processes. You may or may not be open to this, and you may find me off the edge a little bit. But most of the woo woo is in this first chapter just so that you know that I am a spiritual being. I am greater than just a body; I am a being and deeply connected to each of you. We are the oneness no matter if you get that or not. So hold on to your heart chakra, and open up to the knowing of who and what you are. It isn't fear, it isn't guilt, and it isn't shame. You are loved, and loveable. What more can you ask for, what more can you choose, what more can you be? That is up to you and your physical body to decide.

Like many of you, the days have come where I am just so tired of what I am seeing day in and day out scrolling through my newsfeed, and looking through my emails. It is all about the perfect body, the perfect image, the perfect business, and how you can create it all if you just duplicate this plan. It is about judging yourself against the happy people on the other side of those photos. Don't all of the posts and the emails start to sound the same? How many times can you get an "Oops, wrong link" email and actually believe that it's true? And can I just say, "Girl, please!" We all use some sort of filter or another to make the photos look better even if it's just the swiped filter on the Facebook camera. Let yourself open up to the dream of being this amazing you, because that is magic!

Do you know what it's like to feel empty while being successful? It is why I don't duplicate well when someone tells me this is how I have to do something. If you follow Bank Codes you probably know that as woo woo as I am, I like blueprints, but I am in it for action. I am a 'climb out there on the stage and do it my way' type of person. I highly recommend learning what type of being you are so that you know what will drive you to success. Give me a blueprint understanding of why something works; don't just tell me to do it. That is why I like the science behind micronutrients.

A few years back my word for the year was fearless. I tried to take that and turn it around, trying to get beyond my own struggles and connect with others. I have never been the kid that won a popularity contest, because for me it felt like you're being thrust into this black hole, and it just sucks your being out of you. Or maybe that is just my story that I had created to keep me from opening up. Either way, I don't like being told what to do, and I don't like telling people how to do it. We are all the same energy, and yet due to genetics, environment, emotional baggage, we are all vastly different.

So my freedom was to start releasing that grasp on the rigidity, give you the knowledge and let you find your flow.

So I carried this new understanding of flow and move that forward in this book. Rather than tell you how to duplicate my plan, I wanted to stop with the shaming emotions, and the life sucking energy that takes all of the joy out of your desire to just do good things in the world. I want you to drill into what your story is, and figure out how to be in that independent truth. This book is just about speaking the truth of my journey, releasing that knowledge so you can sort through your own history, and gain ideas to actually create a spark of hope that you can find the answers. You can take the ideas, clear off your plate for a month or not. Because in truth, this is your opportunity to throw caution to the wind and start asking your body, "What is going on?"

In 2015 is when I started to question myself a little, and I changed up my wellness program and threw out the rules that my best selling ND author had given to me to follow. I remember driving in the car that one day I told you about, not long after moving into my own path, and just suddenly feeling this moment of clarity where I said, "I'm happy." I hadn't been happy apparently for a very long time. It still catches me off guard some days to just stop and think that I. Am. Happy.

When I suddenly felt happy I asked myself, "What am I doing that I can do more of?" Well for one, it was time to start questioning the status quo that I was living. The questions kept coming and I thought, "What am I learning that I can and should share with others?" I was sure although we are all uniquely different, and yet energetically the same.

Then I dug deeper into, "What can I eliminate from my life to leave a space for what I am being called to do?" Definitely this was easy. There are no rules. I gave up green juice for years because I was told that it was all sugars and no fiber, and would spike my insulin levels. For me that couldn't be further from the truth. I love green juice and if a day goes by that I don't have any, it is a sad day in my body. Recently we had what we joking call 'snowmegeddon' here in Seattle. When we get an inch of snow we close everything down. My favorite cold pressed juice store was closed and I finally braved the break in the storm to get produce and juice for myself. Yes, I will pay more for convenience, but that is how important my green juice is to me. For me it is a vital part of my journey. Finding your vital items will be essential to creating your inner happiness.

I also wanted to ask myself, "What would it take for me to find my destiny?" You know it is so funny to see popular doctor, after popular doctor coin their terms for paleo vegan, and yet never has one reached out to ask me what it is like.

What my friends enjoy about it, how we have modified it, or what caused us to move into the Paleo Vegeo world in the first place. They don't care to know, but that is why I keep sharing that part of my world. I am in my destiny when it comes to this way that I eat, and I refuse to let anyone tell me that I am doing it wrong. I came to this as a quest to find my personal nutritional truth, and so I have and will continue to. What your nutritional truth is may be completely different. The secret is to keep asking until you know what that truth is.

After writing and releasing my "Exploring Aromatherapy" book, I started to work on this new book and I was searching to continue my deeper connection. That book was about teaching people to use oils safely and to use them to enhance their lives. I have spent a lot of time in this life searching for those areas that enhance our lives simply. All of this helps me to understand my inner calling of weirdness. Weirdness tribe, rise up and be heard!

I never seem to be right in the thick of the popularity trends, but a little to the left. I have had my opportunities to create my own private labels, but I don't want to have a chain tugging around with me on this journey to wellness. I love seeking out those items that are true nutrition, ah the joys of non-gmo, and so because of that I get to choose who I open my partnership with and when I am going to take a break from the sales pitch. If it were my own product line, the sales pitch would go on and on forever. That just isn't me. So while I do have products that I highly recommend, I want you to know that it isn't about making a million dollars, it is about truth and the vibrations that come with any product I feel connected about to share with you in this book or elsewhere.

Who I am, and what calls to me really all comes back to what our beings have always known, as highly expansive and highly vibrational. For me it's in the nutrients and how they are facilitated by our body. These body processes are truly what allows us to connect our soul desires to our physical body and feel the joy, climb the mountains, and find the possibilities to do more. When that aligns, our energy is connected to every receptor in our body and we find the spaces in life where we can create the most amazing vitality, and open up to what we are really here to do, build connections and help others.

When I started to shift this change from my first nutritional book, I opened the door to energy healing, quantum biofeedback, meditation, slower living, and self-love and how that facilitates loving others. I had to share all of this with you. This is the magical door for you to open. This is your opportunity to find your "happy". I know that you want it as much as I did.

As I said, I do that "word of the year" thing, and after I shifted my next word of the year had merged from freedom to brilliance. Brilliance can be in the knowledge or it can be in the shine of something you are called for to create. I found this was such a simple shift, and life started to lead me and show me rather than me trying to push down the doors.

When I proofread my last book and this one I was like, "Wow, I am one majorly connected goddess!" I know that I haven't written these books on my own. You cannot open up to this energy awakening just by shining a few beams of light into your soul. It really takes being in the moment and that opens you up to your next creation. Have you ever had this rush of energy that surged through your body, the excited feeling in your stomach as the butterflies start to move, and a deep exhale that releases all of the fear of where you are going? Well I hope as you read through this, it starts to spark that ... because that feeling is mind blowing! When it happened to me all I could see in front of me was my future self in a distant future dancing in emotions, feeling happier and healthier than I have ever been in the shining sun and this amazing group of healers all around me.

I couldn't believe my eyes...
This was something big.

I realized that I've spent most of my life doing things that were safe, not doing things that were empowering and expansive. Fear asks you for safe choices. Joy asks you to let go of limitations, open up to your own path and empower your choices now rather than later. In the past I have let my dreams be overtaken by others, and I just decided no more. I am a seer and I tend to help move others along. The great part about that is that I have amazing sisters in this industry beside me, and I want success for every one of them.

As I connected with this new community and new purposes, my body was changing up my beliefs. This journey opened up more intuitive healing than I thought I could offer. Did you know we are all intuitive? This gift of opportunity is something that I will never overlook, because it's created something divine.

The next year became "transform", and the next year "shift"... and I shifted into healing my wounds. It is a necessary part of the healing process, but you have to be aware that it can be the hardest part of your journey. Taking a new approach to eating, I promise you that once you get it, this will be the easy part. Opening up old wounds and healing them can bring you into a darkness that resurfaces old habits, and old eating habits, old body routines, old emotions as well. As you rise up into that energy, you are going to want this strong micronutrient foundation to stand upon.

Of course, with all of the shifting my 2019 word was "connect" because it was clear that I am meant to keep connecting the dots, keep sharing these sparks of truth with you all, and create something more with all of you. I was meant to connect with something special in 2019 that would change everything about me. Smile and know that when you connect with that energy, time doesn't even exist in the way that you now know it. I want you to know that there is no ending, and you can begin again any time you feel connected to the light. After all your average person changes careers over five times in their lifetime, so why couldn't it be that you are finding a purpose and creating the best you possible you today? Why can't you find your true nutritional path today? Why can't you find the love of your life right now at whatever age you are? Endings are impossible once you learn about quantum physics, and so just open up to the next and the next, and the next. This is exactly what micronutrients actually do. They connect those messenger pathways in your body and open you up to the next possibility, and the next, and the next.

Possibility is always available if you just ask, and the only question is, are you going to answer? How many of you are going to start looking through your back story, start asking questions about the nutrients in your life, and start working with that vagus nerve to find out how much it will change in your body and for you happiness factor?

I want to extend the possibility to talk. One on one communication with someone can help you see where you need an impact in your life. Maybe it's nutrients; maybe it's just one more spark to open you up to ideas. I know that so many crave this as I did, and so now this could be your sign to go forward. Start with joining my group, and I will connect and add you to learn, and share with healers, dreamers and doers. Our focus is simple. Nutritional brilliance is energy. Dreaming about something lighter and lifting each other to create changes that impact generations in a healthier direction.

So if you have a lot of digestive work, both physically and mentally after reading this intro, believe that this is because you are seeing that spark to find your personal plan, by letting go of the limitations of everything you have been told you have to do. The only thing we are required to do in this life to stay alive is be, breathe, sleep, drink water and eat food. How you take those tasks on is what will change the course of your future.

My target in this world is to create higher vibrations through elevated nutrition and consciousness. I feel like this book can help others set that foundation. Please let me know what it offers to you. Until then I am going to move deeper into my work with energy, working with my heart, and see what else I can choose for this life. I invite you to join me.

2

Dominoes & Details

It all starts so very simple, and yet it can domino before you realize what has happened. That is exactly how it happened to me and has happened to you. This book is my story, and it's my journey to wellness. I know it says epigenetics in the foreword quote, but that is a never ending journey. Epigenetics is the process of gene expression. Genes can be turned on, and genes can be turned off. Thankfully it's one that items you can learn from and pass along to the next generation.

All real change happens because we're open to the possibility for something more. I have always believed in something more, and in creating a world of greater vibrations. I believe that nutrition can and will elevate your consciousness. I believe that micronutrients facilitate body processes. I believe that we were built with receptors because we were meant to receive, and that opens up choices. Some of those choices can block out what we desire and cut us off from harmony. It's a domino effect and only we can make a different choice. Some of us will have to go back to our beginnings, but most of us will have to go back further and rewrite everything we think we are, and everything we think we know. You can call it belief clearing, or you epigenetic expression. Either way we need to acknowledge that this started generations ago, and compounded.

You existed in the growing body of your mother when she was in your grandmother's womb. How's that for mind blowing? I am one of the many that have accepted that I was created before I was even a thought, and I am releasing the inner toxic landmines so that future generations will have better choices. I am still rewriting this story daily, and so are you. Try to remember that when one door closes, another door or window is opening and so that this is not about one right answer, it is about listening for the harmony in your own story.

My life story, I thought, started when I was born prematurely. I felt like an only child when I was a toddler because I was the first girl, and had no close sibling like my Irish twin brothers did. When my sister did come along it was an annoyance more than anything for both of us. She crossed my face out in photos with big sharpie markers, she was dressed like me, and she had all of daddy's love and affection. I felt that I was the carbon copy, although I came first. How funny that I later learned she and I both felt this same emotional baggage, when in reality we were and are so very different in personality. So while she also felt like she was my carbon copy, in reality we looked so much alike that people often thought we were twins. She was taller, and genetically thinner than I was. I was more active, and genetically more of a lone wolf than she was. That lone worth personality too has flipped in our adulthood as I am now more social and she is a homebody.

One of my first memories after she was born was staring into the hospital window at her and my mom. I think I tried to disconnect from that relationship almost immediately. I can remember later I would sit outside on the grass on those bright summer days far away from anyone that might burst my personal bubble. My sister couldn't go into the sun or the grass because it would cause a horrible rash, so this was my escape. A sun allergy is an immune system reaction to sunlight and she had a horrible immune system as a child, and this was another thing we had shared in different ways but at similar ages in our childhood.

Out there in the sunshine is where that first sign showed up that I could later trace to being the first toxic secret link. It's also where hers probably got continually worse because of the lack of natural vitamin D she was missing out on. At the time I was probably in kindergarten or first grade and I spent as many sunny days outside in the grass, or hiding behind the grape vines eating all of those grand, organic polyphenols I could get my hands on. When I needed even more of a cave to escape to, those grape vines were my harbor in the storm.

I can remember sitting in the yard that summer being that joyful energy on this grass island where no sister could venture. My sister would stare at me, probably wishing to venture into my arena of happiness, as she played under the carport with the cats. The truth is that the cats probably instinctively wanted exactly what I had. We are part juicy energy, and part animal. Our lizard brain instinct is there to help us in so many ways, and yet they are also the items we most overlook as we stumble into this world of trying to figure out our bodies. We don't think about what our bodies are, how they function, or even how they heal until we are in a moment of scarcity due to disease and gene expressions that create chaos in our life.

Animals will lick a wound and rarely you will see little kids doing the same. It is a lizard brain reaction to remove debris and speed up healing. Have you ever tasted blood and thought, "What is this!?" Blood has that copper taste, and although we aren't vampires many people are literally addicted to copper. You aren't really tasting copper, but the metallic components of our red blood cells, but metals can be highly addictive to those with high histamine and low adrenal function.

When I was little I was one that routinely could be found getting in trouble for roaming around with a penny in my mouth. Of course pennies are just coated with copper, and so there was no supplementation going on, just a tick on the timeline. There is no such thing as a week without chocolate at my house. Did you know that chocolate is high in copper? We know that there is a possibility of copper deficiency weakening the immune system, which can cause people to get sick more often. Copper is the most abundant trace mineral in the human body. However copper toxicity also messes with zinc metabolism, and that impacts our immune system as well. I personally believe I have had a long term problem with copper toxicity, and a craving for more. You don't have to eat high copper to be copper toxic; it can just be that your body is not properly metabolizing it. Many of the genetic codes we are now working with are just improperly metabolizing micronutrients, and generally the more synthetic it is the more likely to struggle with metabolizing it.

I didn't know for most of my childhood that genetics play an important role in who we are beyond looking like our family, not that environment can change our DNA. What I did know about myself early on, I can intuitively tune in and help others. My belief is that we can all tune in, but some of us just don't choose to do so. There is no wrong energy when it comes to our energetic inner self. How many of those with that inner knowing almost always refuse to tune in to anything that is related to your own well-being? (Looks out across the sea of all of you empathic and intuitive beings raising their hands.)

Interestingly enough, 2017 was a breakthrough year for me in terms of acceptance and truth of this gift as the synchronicities kept stacking up. The more I asked, the more I opened up. It was more than manifesting a car, although I did get the SUV that I put up on my vision board without realizing it. Every day now I am still surprised that I ask, and the universe offers, even though I know that is exactly how it works. We tune in, and what we desire we become aware of.

The last few years have been all about tuning into me as much as I tuned into others. So I sat down to start sorting out my own wellness and realized if I go back in time to the first moments that I remember my body trying to tell me my story, it goes back not just to those summer days, but to generations before my birth. My body was telling me tiny stories that were parts of underlying DNA mutations related to the functional pathways in my body. Now I am a listener, and now I am a belief clearer and energy transmutator (is that a real word?). My hope is that you will learn through going through this book to listen to your own story, and create something completely elevated.

The most talked about genetic mutation of the last decade is the variety of the MTHFR mutations. If you Google "MTHFR" there are about 1,700,000 results. Everyone I have tested in my family has at least one MTHFR variation, and not all the same variation. It runs in our family along with the other 25% of the population. This knowledge showed that both my mother and my husband's mother have the same MTHFR mutation, and the same as my daughter. So mine comes from another DNA source. With my father being dead and my brothers not taking a DNA test, I can only guess that the other comes from my father.

If you have a MTHFR mutation and start down the rabbit hole you will find this genetic alteration is notorious for causing high heavy metals in the system. These heavy metals in our system become harder to be broken down properly, and are instead stored. This storage can cause a list of symptoms including fatigue, which is usually the first signal. The hardest part for us to realize is that these heavy metals are passed down generationally. So what your ancestors several generations were absorbing becomes yours. Those metal amalgams full of mercury and other metals are passed into the brains of our children in the womb. I had six cavities to be filled at age five, and I cringed thinking about this after having my daughter.

When my daughter was a year old I craved the naps we took together. It was more than the deep postpartum depression that I had for a year and a half. Even though my next door neighbor had anemia, I didn't put it together for myself. Yes, you can have high heavy metals and low iron stores. When you have a high heavy metal in your system it starts to impact many areas of your functional system. One of those can be brain fog. Of course motherhood also gives you a little brain fog, so we don't always think anything of it.

Our kids come home from school tired after drinking heavy metal toxic water all day, and we don't think anything of that either. One interesting thing about a heavy metal like copper is that you crave more copper because it stimulates your fatigued brain. So we crave that which is doing us harm because we need it, or sometimes just needing it in a more bioavailable form. Think of it as the person with chronic gastric issues that can't stay away from caffeine despite what it's doing to their gut.

When my daughter was an infant I also didn't know a lot about micronutrients. Since then I have learned that selenium can form inactive complexes with heavy metals which can further enhance their detoxification, and I didn't know that there are several types of selenium to choose from. Of course if you live in the UK you have pretty much zero selenium in your soil. (4) Farming practices also tend to disrupt our nutrients in the soil, and thus we start lacking some nutrients and through commercial farming getting too much of others. In more recent studies it has been found that infants are at risk of selenium deficiency, especially true in the breastfed baby. Taking in a small amount of selenium rich food can give an infant what it needs as breast milk responds to organic and inorganic selenium in the mom's whole foods and supplementation.

Glyphosate, the most common of all herbicides used across the globe for commercial farming, also disrupts selenium uptake in plants and to me that seems very unhelpful to the 25% of the United States population with the MTHFR mutated genes eating the standard American diet. This may be a part of the puzzle on why we are seeing a rise in autoimmune diseases like Hashimoto's and Celiac disease. As well, consider that the number of kids being diagnosed on the spectrum keeps rising, and has its own link to parental autoimmune disorders. A large scale study in Denmark showed high increased risks for having a child on the spectrum when one parent had an autoimmune disorder. Not so shocking then that many children on the spectrum also have been shown to usually have an increased copper serum level.

All of this excess copper can do a number on a system that isn't performing in a 'normal' manner including depleting essential nutrients like vitamin C, zinc and folate, just as an example. So when your body craves folate, and you aren't getting anything but synthetic sources that just sit in the folate receptor, it is creating a cycle that stops facilitation in the body across the methylation pathway, and reducing the fuel for your endocrine system. Our bodies create an excess of so many metals like copper, and even methylmercury. In turn the pituitary gland and other glands do not get what they want, like the adrenals. The pituitary gland is responsible for releasing prolactin. Prolactin works with lactation, and how many women struggle with lactation. My daughter wouldn't latch, and I wasn't producing what she required, anyway. Prolactin is also responsible for keeping our dopamine in check. Prolactin can create a negative feedback loop with dopamine production and impacts our happy state of serotonin.

Extensive evidence that we now have shown that serotonin is a neuroendocrine controller that works within the body to support the regulation of the secretion of several pituitary hormones. On top of that there are many reproductive dysfunctions that are now believed to be associated with elevations of prolactin. This is one heck of a multipurpose hormone. Heavy metals are prolactin disruptors and many of the items that we would see in a body when there is an increase or decrease of the prolactin released, you also see in a body when there is too much heavy metal build up. Why aren't we talking about heavy metals?

I was recently listening to a doctor talk about areas that were impacted by his own high levels of mercury. However, he found that it wasn't the mercury or copper, but perhaps lead that was fueling his problems. He shared with us how his lead levels and his son's levels were very high, yet they had never been exposed to lead in their home. Heavy metals, the gift from your grandparents that you never asked for. Thanks so much, genetics and ancestry for all that you give, without a roadmap to help us through the dark and dank forest. The forest is both a gift and a hot mess. Not everyone is open to figuring out their mess, but eventually they will be hit with it head on.

Did you know that having elevated levels of the heavy metals lead and cadmium can result in an increased incidence of asthma, as demonstrated in recently published research from Brown University? (18) These heavy metals cause a shift in our TH1/TH2 response and then lead to much greater production of IgE, the allergic antibody that causes asthma. Where most of our generational cadmium comes from is cigarette use and work in the mines. Miners, like my Grandfather, were exposed to and in turn exposed their families to cadmium. They have finally said that there is first hand, second hand a third hand cigarette smoke. This third hand is the invisible tobacco dust that settles in the environment and stays there even after a cigarette has been put out. This dust contains more than 250 chemicals. We are all at risk of exposure to these types of heavy metals and other damaging, toxic chemicals.

If you follow me you know that I created what is called the Paleo Vegeo lifestyle over a decade ago. I did this because I was vegan and wanted to try paleo, but the only answers online were that you could not do that. Over the years I have learned that a lot of the paleo teachings need to be unlearned, but I have also learned a lot about nutrition and veganism. A lot of healthy vegans are exposed to cadmium through rice and cereal grains grown in ion contaminated soils. Brown rice is not just hard to digest, but it is heavily toxic most of the time. I prefer dull, overly processed, white rice as a resistant starch rather than as a healthy food option.

These chemicals are also in the tap water we drink, and unlike copper or zinc and a few others, cadmium is not essential to our bodies. We store this cadmium, like some other toxins, in our kidneys and the liver. Urinary cadmium excretion is a very slow process, and unfortunately is our major mechanism for elimination.

Cadmium accumulates in our bodies over a lifetime and its biologic half-life may be up to 38 years. For those that don't know what this means, the biologic half-life is how long a substance (for example a metabolite, drug, signaling molecule, radioactive nuclide, or other substance) takes to lose half of its pharmacologic, physiologic, or radiologic activity. That's a long time!! How many of you had a child before the age of 38? How many of you started feeling really, really bad by the time you were 40?

Unlike cadmium, which settles in and stores up, copper is a wanderer, and also a needed element we need for life. You can't live without copper, even though copper is a systemic trouble maker in your life. Copper can circulate freely in our body, and it accumulates not just in the liver, but also primarily in the brain and female organs. Everything that doesn't metabolize properly first impacts the liver. Keep that in mind as you continue to read through this journey. Copper is also an endocrine disrupting metal, and yet as I said, we need it. It is essential to the proper functioning of our immune system, the same endocrine system it can disrupt, and our nervous system. It is so unfortunate that copper can quickly get out of balance and create complications in all three of those areas.

Without copper functioning properly, I found that my body was less likely to be able to control the bad guys in my gut and we know how important this area is to many areas of our wellness. There is a whole realm of research based on the now known HPA Axis (hypothalamic-pituitary-adrenal axis). Copper imbalance also doesn't always mean you have a body that cannot use copper. It can also show that you are deficient, or that your body is a very smart planner. When you have a lot of copper in the body, it will start to increase the sodium levels. However the smart body says it needs to retain copper in order to shore itself up from the impact if you have continual issues like stress as these two are partners in crime.

So many children and adults today have low immune systems, and low serotonin disorders, and histamine intolerance, adhd, and on and on. It is time for us to realize that minerals are impacted by pollutants just as much as in this very minute as one hundred years ago. We live in a time when just as many children and adults have leaky guts, and protein reactions that aren't being explained. We keep seeing "allergies" in people that have never had these problems before. We are seeing an epidemic in depression and suicide. What we are seeing is the microbiome generation. By that I mean those without the healthy microbiota community to be the healing warriors for our body. We are our gut, and our gut is our environmental trigger for this unwanted epigenetic process.

Of course when you are born via C-section your gut isn't at its best to begin with. One in three children born today is born via C-section. I know that there is a lot of talk about how C-section bypasses the vaginal microbiota transfer; however I was additionally in the hospital as a preemie for some time. I was dealt the blow of antibiotics during childhood followed by strange bacterial immunology shots as a child. I have now followed the paper trail that shows that copper toxicity can be connected to Staphylococcus aureus (1) and I have figured out that it is very much a part of my puzzle.

Many immunosuppressive heavy metals, like copper and mercury, are associated with infectious diseases, and heavy metal tests in immunosuppressed individuals are often quite high. Even before the summers of copper love, I had dealt with S. aureus for a long, long time. S. aureus is often found on a mother's nipples, and almost as often as in her nostrils. Looking at the stool of infants researchers often find S. aureus strains, and 90% are identical to the parental skin strain. There is no competition to this strain, and so it's no wonder that researchers in Sweden found that 60% of the infants had S. aureus strains in the stools, even though only 24% of their mothers did. These heavy metals serve as a source of food for viruses, bacteria, parasites, and other pathogens like these in our body, and it's more complex if you don't have the microbiome from a vaginal birth to fight it.

My mother loves telling me the story of how adorable it was to see me run about the house with a bare bottom. I have always had what she termed a "bubble butt". However the truth is, she first started letting me go diaper-less because I had a large boil on my bottom when I was learning to walk. As I said before, Staphylococcus aureus is very common in infants. Research currently shows staph and it's more serious variety MRSA infections are also becoming more common in children every year.

Staphylococcus aureus, or staph, was first identified in Scotland in the 1880's. It wasn't until the 1930's that there was any sort of test to diagnose staph in wounds. Because of the outbreak of staph infections they were deliberately colonizing infants with the S. aureus. There is no way for me to know at this time what the cause of my boil was, or the reasons I was given shots weekly over a number of years after having that boil. Those shots didn't stop until my mom forced the doctors to wean me off of the shots. The medical facilities where I was treated are long gone, so I have no idea if I was given gamma-globulin shots like others were for their low immune system, or long-term antibiotic therapy, or maybe even something completely different. Regardless of the type of treatment I received, I am sure it had an additional impact on my microbiome that has continued through my entire life. I also am sure that the early S. aureus exposure is another domino in my life issues.

Before reading this did you know that when you are born you can be born with staph, or even another infection, as well as these heavy metals? Just like these heavy metals, there are several infections that can pass from mother to child including Lyme, fungus (yeast) and/or candida, and C. diff to name a few. People often say that they cannot figure out where they picked this disease up, and yet it often just goes right back home through our parents and many more generations deep. Similarly parents feed baby, and they pass the bad bacteria from their mouth to baby's mouth or from breast to babes as soon as they are born.

Candida albicans and Staphylococcus aureus are often co-isolated in cases of biofilm-associated infections. (3) A biofilm is a thin, slimy film of bacteria, and comprises any group of microorganisms where the cells stick to each other or to a surface. Bacterial biofilms are triggers, and yet they are a genetically-driven process in our body. I think there is a biological reason that lactoferrin is fed to infants via breastmilk, and that lactoferrin helps prevent bacterial biofilm development. Of course I know this now, and had a child who refused to breastfeed no matter what I did. I was in the hospital for so long, eerily similar to my mom's birth, I often wonder how much formula supplementation I received. What part of what we are given at birth, or not given at birth creates the reactions to our own bodies, and how does our body remember? Is there something in the breast milk that is protective against staph and other bacteria that creates a memory in our immune system to fight it later in life?

Our immune system has memory T-cells, and these are the cells of the immune system that make antibodies to invading pathogens like viruses. They are called this because they form memory cells that remember the same pathogen for faster antibody production in future infections. These are the same memory cells that I now fight against in my personal mast cell war. I no longer test allergic to many items when they skin test me, however my body remembers those offenders and defend itself it must! Most of the T-cell memory is formed in the first 5 years of life, and this is the reasoning that I have been given for why children are given so many vaccines in the first few years of life. I personally think that we are on the brink of some very important discoveries on being able to generate new memory T-cells to fight off infections and disease in an entirely different way.

My sister was also one of those that had shots for a very long time when we were little, after I was done with my odd inoculations. Her shots were not weekly, but were monthly and we were told it was just because she had a low immune system. I had German measles five times when I was little, and my sister had chicken pox at least as many times. I remember being thrilled that she was getting a shot, which meant I would get an ice cream at the pharmacy. I remember these dominos, and I am sure our bodies do as well.

Her story, or dominos, however does not start there. Long before the shots and ice cream, my sister had these odd seizures. They came and went between 10 months and a year old, grand mal seizures. The first was when we were hiking above my uncle's home in the foothills of the Wasatch Mountains. I cannot even imagine what my mom went through in those moments running her baby down the mountain to get her to the hospital, all while fearing her daughter was going to die. Now we start to come full circle back to my first secret clue.

I have seen at least one study that showed a connection between high serum copper in children with unprovoked seizures where they had normal MRI scan and abnormal EEG. (2) She hasn't had a seizure since, however she had to overcome learning disabilities that our pediatrician believed was connected to those early seizures she suffered with. Maybe it wasn't copper, maybe it was it a diabetic seizure caused by low blood sugar. Maybe it was a seizure brought on by mitochondrial dysfunction? Or maybe she has a magnesium disorder because she still cannot take magnesium in any sort of supplement without getting very ill, similarly to my daughter. We're still not sure, however seeing my family's genetics as we have all gotten tested, I do have my suspicions. I do know that her body, just like all of our bodies do, was telling a story. We all are being told stories and yet we don't wake up to it until we are so far in, it is hard to dig out. Now in her 40's she is dealing with the clean-up, which is part of my reason for delving into this subject. Families are dealing with these toxic scenarios and nutrient disorders in greater numbers than we have ever seen before. It is like unraveling a thread on a much loved sweater. If you keep unraveling you will get to that first stitch.

The first stitch for me was a book by Dr. William J. Walsh called 'Nutrient Power'. This book was about the five biotypes that he has classified by nutrients that are overloading the body, as well as those that a person may be deficient in. When talking about genetic mutations you will often hear someone discuss their undermethylation or overmethylation problems. There is a lot of information out there to sort through while trying to become your own methylation guru. He has helped me understand more of what was happening to my daughter when her eosinophil count was through the roof when tested. The assumption was Mast Cell disorder, which he has shown goes hand in hand with methylation imbalances. We were doing everything we could to strengthen her mast cells, but without the proper functioning, it was just a Band-Aid on the problem, and the problem was just a symptom.

Methylation can be understood like a team working towards an end project. Each member of the team has a job to do in order to complete it. When a system is undermethylated there may be a team member that is hoarding rather than passing on the job. Phosphatidylcholine is something that is talked a lot about, and is the major membrane phospholipid in our cells. As an example it is a very important constituent of our lipoproteins, lung surfactant and bile. Choline can appear in food in many forms besides phosphatidylcholine (also known as lecithin), but also as free choline, sphingomyelin, glycerophosphocholine, and phosphocholine. Over 50% of your methylation reactions involve these phospholipids, and some people also have genetic mutations that make conversion complicated. People often think that if you don't eat eggs, you are missing out on the benefits of choline. Vegans that eat gently (and freshly) ground flaxseeds see their phospholipids incorporated into the cell membranes of our body. As well, cruciferous vegetables are one of the richest sources of phosphatidylcholine, the principle phospholipid our cell membranes need, although not great for everyone in large amounts.

Synchronicities, they seem to sew my life together as I have gotten older. When I was younger I wanted so badly to move to Seattle, and then there was a job that I felt my husband was perfect for and sent off his resume, of course without telling him I had. He got that job and we spent some beautifully chaotic years there. However, I wanted to move back to Utah to be near family and have a baby, and everything fell into place just as easily. The same week my husband's contract was up, so was our lease on our apartment. The following week he had a contract to start in Utah. Like I said, many synchronicities.

After having my daughter, and slowly taking some changes to my lifestyle, I found the book, 'The Veganist', which I am sure I was meant to find. I went vegan after doing a 21 Day Vegan Kickstart. This took place long before I learned about epigenetics, but it just felt right. Recently I found out that I am genetically more inclined to have a heart attack because my flat, sticky little blood platelets do exactly what comes natural to them and stick together. So before I knew that plants were my medicine, I knew I felt better eating more plants. What are you being told that you aren't listening to? If you believe that we are being given information that we are supposed to use and share, then energetically this was meant to happen for me and it will happen for you.

So because of the synchronicities of life, I gratefully elevated my awareness. I am always watching for what information I need to know like a unicorn hawk. Listen, that could happen. A big one regarding my daughter was going to an evening event with Robyn Openshaw in a small town called North Bend, WA just after we moved back to Seattle. The day after that event I took my daughter off all dairy, and five weeks later off all of her daily inhaled steroids. Synchronicities. Three years ago as I was deep into tweaking my methylation pathways, a friend took me to an evening event to listen to an enthusiastic, young ND from California speak about nutrition. That night was another one of those life changing sync ups.

Listening to this NorCal ND five years after taking my daughter off daily steroids I leaned into a big change with our supplementation and switched to an encapsulated whole foods program. This, I believe, is what eliminated the six times a year steroid dump where she would be on oral steroids for three days at a time. My daughter grew two inches in six months after we made that switch, and then stopped having that croup five to six times per year. I feel blessed every day that I listened to what I knew we needed.

Recently the next pathway opened for me in this journey as I started exploring more dietary changes. I realized that the least mitochondria and oxidative supportive plants are: Avocados, Bananas, Figs, Grapefruits, Pineapple, Bok Choy, Brussels sprouts, Cabbage, Carrots, Cauliflower, Cucumbers, Endive, Mushrooms, Peppers (sweet red and green), Potatoes (white or yellow), Pumpkin, Spinach, Squash (yellow), Tomatoes and Zucchini. So I looked at the foods I was regularly eating, and I thought... well that is just rude!! These foods were my jam! Am I right? These were the foods that I lived for. I sort of cried a little inside when I thought about this. Cauliflower is joy if you are paleo and vegan, and avocado, even though I can't eat it due to my latex hypersensitivity.

The Summer of 2018 my mast cells let me know they were tired of whatever it was that was bothering them, and I know a lot of what that is tied to. When it happened I told myself it was just a keto rash as I was in deep into my Ketolicious Reset program, but as I got worse it was apparent that keto rash is just a term we are giving to mast cell reactivity. When you start to ask the questions, and really want the answers, they will start to show up in your life like magic. They aren't always in the form you desire, but they will show up.

Synchronicity... it abounds around us. When you least expect it to happen, everything you need will show up. Try to watch and listen to what it's telling you, write down notes when you hear something in this book that lights you up. The goal as you go through my stories should be to learn to be more aware of the synchronicities in your life. Take a short time to reflect and write down some items that stick out about your childhood that may be those details you missed in figuring out your wellness journey.

I do eat cucumbers almost daily, and today they are sliced thinly in my miso soup. Yet awareness was telling me to listen to this new idea, and I did. This idea of change after a decade of teaching and sharing the Paleo Vegeo lifestyle was something my body seemed to be pulling me towards. I am guessing that many of you reading all of this and seeing a similar picture to your own path, now is the time to reset your own story. I ask you to leave aside your judgements, stop creating beliefs, and just let your path unfold like magic.

3

Dietary Fads

Myself, as I was deeply listening to my inner guides after the long year of learning called 2017, I started my group's January Paleo Vegeo Whole30 Vegan 2018 challenge. I had a good friend jump in to start the challenge with me. As I watched her follow all of the rules, I started to see this Whole30 program through her eyes. It was extreme and she lost weight in a very unhealthy manner. She wasn't vegan, but vegetarian. Like many of the lazy keto followers she was eating loads of eggs, avocado, and very low micronutrient balance. It sort of lit this fire under me to start looking at what I was teaching others. Here I was running what is still the largest paleo vegan group on Facebook for vegan, vegetarian or pescatarian followers, and I was tired of what it was creating. I was also so tired of the three-quarters of a page that the paleo community was giving to what I felt was the key to changing our bodies from the inside out. I started this as a purpose to get others to find their own personalized nutrition plan, and here I was living in the same sad sandbox as everyone else. Do you know what cats do in sandboxes? It was an eye opening moment and so I took a leap of faith into trying to sort out what mattered most in our dietary challenge.

I started the year with a blaze, because don't we all? I changed my diet and started allowing non-gmo soy back into my life for the first time in almost 20 years, and in the first 6 weeks I lost 8 pounds. That is a huge number for me now that I am in menopause. When you get there ladies (and gentlemen) the weight doesn't seem to always move in the direction you desire. I was eating a lot of those unhelpful plants though, and I was feeling it. I also added in more fats. Everything I read says that ketogenic, low-carb dieting is what menopausal women need. I plugged my DNA into one of those diet companies and it also says that I should eat a lower carb diet. Who doesn't want to jump on the high fat bandwagon? I am one of those that kept trying it again, and again, and again. Every time I gained weight and always ended up feeling awful. I finally decided this time that it had to be the high saturated fats combined with my low functioning adrenals. But what else could it be?

Since I am a biohacker, I decided I just needed to adjust to high monounsaturated fats and the initial creation of the Ketolicious Reset was born. Even though this other nutritional nudge kept coming into my vision that had nothing to do with how many fats I was eating, I kept going for the fats. In my practice I have worked with more people with gastroparesis in the past two years than you can imagine. This little talked about disorder has a variety of issues that it is connected to, but I was really afraid when my body wasn't digesting the way it always had in the past. I suffered my first gallbladder attack in my life the first week of February, and boy was it the most painful thing ever. As vegans we don't consider the gallbladder because it must just be acid reflux. However there is more to if for those of us with autoimmune genetics than we have been told. If you Google "gallbladder" or "sluggish bile" you are told to take bile salts most often. However, these bile salts have potent detergent properties and can have damaging effects on our cell membranes. If we go back to phospholipids in the cell membranes, then it's important to know that along with betaine, which is it's metabolite; phosphatidylcholine functions as a methyl donor. Methylation issues anyone??

Other rich sources of choline are soy products, quinoa, and broccoli. If you have followed me for years you know that I am not a fan of quinoa because of the damage it's doing to the soil in the countries where most of it is grown, the gluten that often comes along with it as a ride-along, and the fact that the saponins it contains when eaten along with dietary cholesterol, interferes with the absorption by forming an insoluble complex. It also will form insoluble complexes with minerals, such as zinc and iron, which make the minerals unavailable for absorption in your gut. Are you iron and zinc deficient? How do you make and eat your quinoa? When I first went vegan I was eating a lot of quinoa. It wasn't until I decided to do a paleo vegan option that I realized just how much I was eating, and the truth that it wasn't doing anything for my body. If the Whole30 has a highlight for coming into my life, it is that elimination can be a beautiful part of figuring out what works and what doesn't.

The change in my diet that I had selected for this "new me" was to increase my fat intake, but I wasn't very careful and it also increased the Omega-6s that I was eating by mega amounts. In my group everyone always has these great recipes using almond butter, or cashew butter, and even sunflower butter. I cannot eat any of those. I generally have used hemp seed butter, but it's so very green that I wanted a change. I found a brand of organic, non-gmo soy butter and it was delicious, and made without sugar with just a little added organic soy oil and sustainable palm oil. This also was added to my diet in large amounts. I was cooking in gobs of coconut oil, so all of this fatty joy increased not just my monounsaturated fats, but my polyunsaturated fats (PUFA) and saturated fats. I was tracking my progress and I was totally in the ketogenic zone. My body just wasn't going to have any of it.

Those PUFA's I found out are linked to thyroid function, which impacts the gallbladder. (5) I have suffered from severe adrenal fatigue for years, which I see running rampant throughout my family. My cortisol spikes in the evening, and makes it hard to sleep if I don't get to bed before that starts. That also means there are some underlying hormone issues, but that part of the equation we can talk more about later. Cortisol, which is released by these crazy adrenals of mine, slows down the function of the thyroid because it has slowed down the hypothalamus and pituitary gland. It is one of those circles of Hell that I think so many of us suffer with.

Now I am going to get a little geeky, and unless you have had thyroid problems you may not understand anything I am saying for a second. The hypothesis was out there, and what they are saying right now is that cytokines, our cell signaling molecules, decrease T3 induction of 5' D-I, resulting in decreased T3 production. (or at least reduced active T3 production) 5' D-I is the enzyme responsible for converting thyroxine, or T4 to T3. What this means is that when you have less active thyroid hormones, you have less energy in every cell in your body. However, what happens when you add low hormones and high inflammation together is a ticking time bomb. The more inflammation, the less those hormone receptors function properly. Inflammation is the most vastly impacting "disease" of our generation.

With adrenal fatigue, initially when the cortisol level is very high, our immune functions are lowered, but the anti-inflammatory cell signals reduce inflammation in the body. So not a lot of pain. So why don't we then do several HIIT workouts a week and feel really good? Sound familiar?

When our adrenals are just done with this stressed out life, they start this major inflammatory cycle by lowering cortisol production. This is where for those of you that have never done well on T4 do better with just a little T3. When adrenals are struggling with low cortisol, they clearly need T3 before chaos happens. Our gut is responsible for a fifth of the T4 to T3 conversion, of course. I am very happy there are more conversations happening and more research going into why we have low T3, rather than just focusing in on T4. For me all of this clarity helped me figure out why it could be so very hard to figure out thyroid functions when you have adrenals running the show. I started thinking very hard about what it could be that was impacting so many people, and yet we are all testing normal. This is when you need to look at your Reverse T3 levels.

It's important to remember that so many of the wellness cycles we're talking about start in the gut, the epicenter of our being. If there is a place where our soul is gently sewn together with our physical bodies, I think it must be in that Solar Plexus region. These muscle friends of ours rely on proper thyroid function. If the sphincter doesn't relax, then bile acid secretion is impaired. Thinking about this process helped me determine part of the reason why I felt the way I did. I realized that my body's thyroid hormone wasn't relaxing my gallbladder's opening, and why after years of eating little to no fat that my bile acid wasn't secreting out to break down these fats. I was suddenly for the first time in decades eating PUFA's, and I wasn't eating enough of the good fatty acids, so my balance was way off. As a long standing vegan that didn't eat many fats, I was not digesting these fats. Beyond that I wasn't getting the minerals I needed. At the end of that first six weeks my gut was unhappier than it had been in years, and my energy being felt it. There is nothing like a group of spiritual guides and your infinite being sitting there together deciding just how much to throw at you when you are not listening to a damn thing.

As you can see with each detail you uncover it becomes a deeper rabbit hole that tips over another domino. So as I have watched where the dominoes have been placed, and what had caused them to fall, I have begun tracking. That's something that is always a key in figuring out what is going on; track what is happening right now. If we don't write things down we often won't remember them later. That causes a stalemate in the wellness struggle, and so we go searching for another supplement, another book, another diet without getting to the root cause. I dug through what I felt was the most influential dietary items that anyone born into this autoimmunity generation can change with ease and that is where I started.

The program I had been using for most of my 40's made me feel like I was being punished for what I wanted to eat. Strictly following "the rules" made me feel like my choices were all wrong. In fact the entire thing made me feel almost embarrassed at how much I love and embraced the multitude of supplements I had started to use, even though they made me feel better than I had for most of my life. Instead of eating 30 plus plants in a capsule, I was being told to eat a specific amount of "perfectly compliant foods" because why? Eating this way meant no low processed soy that I found I still loved. It meant I couldn't enjoy the white rice that has been on my plate multiple times a day when I felt my healthiest about fifteen year prior. That says a lot because that was after I had stopped having daily severe IBD episodes that were completely debilitating. I had to remove a food that my gut loved, and it was about time for me to have a say in my food choices again. We so often wrap ourselves up in the energy of being wrong, that we are the creators of the damages we are facing. As an energy intuitive mama, let me be the first to say that the woo-woo isn't all woo-woo. Read the, 'Biology of Belief' and get back to me.

I have shared a little of those feelings in my private group over the years, but overall I have stuck to the four walls of Paleo within Veganism to lend the support and help those looking to take on this rigid wellness challenge. When I didn't there was a cry from the "believers" that how could I mention tempeh??? Fad diets are like your average network marketing companies. Cults. I expect to see Leah Remini do a special on either the Paleo diet or the Keto diet any week now. The rules are don't eat grains (guess what... lots of misinformation about grains and lectins, phytic acids, etc. out there). Don't eat anything that comes out of a box (expect the bars and salad dressing and other goodies we approve of). Don't eat legumes (despite the fact that Dan Buettner spent over a decade studying the places that people live the longest, and beans were a superfood that can add four years to your life). Do not consume anything that seems like it is food joy (no pancakes, no muffins and of course no homemade pizza for heaven's sake!). What I ended up with is a lot of guilt and shame for cheering people on to deprive themselves. This is the emotion I have been carrying around for years. We hold onto these emotions and they create energy implants that are very hard to shake.

Also, to be quite vulnerable and honest, I felt ashamed every time someone got through the program and they didn't get results, or the weight went right back on. I watched 4,000 people run through my group, with just a handful sharing how this was their diet for life. I worked myself in and out of months of thirty day challenges, and pushing aside the foods that my body really craved. One moment finally brought me to questioning so many things about how we are being TOLD how to sell, how to eat, how to live, how to feel. When the best seller is a book that tells women to lose weight in order to feel successful enough to sell their products, there is a problem with the system. As I changed things up, guess what, you do have to eat some plants every day. Sorry... however I found that every body can be reset. So I got busy figuring out how to share this knowledge so that you can figure your body out, rather than just following another program.

I started a conversation in my group last summer and told them in no uncertain terms that this group come January is changing. My mindset of being in a box is changing. We are curvy, and varied, and all desire to feel well, and find out what works for our own body. If you create an underlying foundation of dense nutrition, you can then move onto the next question for your body, and then the next, and then the next. This last November I spent a month working on digging into the emotions of why we treat our bodies so badly. This focus had to become more grounding, and less shame.

These fad programs are like traditional school. You are a gorgeous and expansive circle being taught to fit in the tiny square hole, rather than being whatever you desire. As a homeschooling hybrid mom this new world is growing by leaps and bounds because we are realizing that we don't want our kids to learn to just work in a factory for fifty years. We want them to learn to be happy, for all of their life (or lives if you go there). So I started looking at how all of the parts of all of our puzzles work together.

I do know real food supplementation, well that has to happen, and it has to start with a true whole food foundation to get your body right. We just use the products that come from nature so much more efficiently than synthetics. I am not embarrassed to say that. Nine times out of ten when I talk to someone that is struggling and we go through their diet and the list is lacking in much needed supplementation. It makes me a little sad to think they are missing out greatly in something that to me was almost like finding the MTHFR enzyme for my genetic mutation in a leafy green. Do you sometimes need the one off "ingredient" vitamin? Sure! But when my male clients are lifting weights they are using suma root, and not steroids, to beef up their lean body mass.

I read this report from Harvard Health recently, and it agreed with what we are seeing today. In the early 1940s no one had measurable levels of folic acid in the bloodstream because all our folate came from food. I just said folic, and not folate. The use of multivitamins and the addition of folic acid to many foods has changed that. A report from the Framingham Heart Study shows that most Americans have some folic acid in their blood, and 20% or more have high levels of it.

So truth, even if you don't have the MTHFR mutation, eating all of those enriched processed foods is giving everyone free range folic acid in their bloodstreams, and sitting waiting to be metabolized in the liver, and so it's not really a mutation problem at all but a processed food problem.

There is also a study that was measuring the methylfolate concentration of seven fruits and vegetables that were rinsed thoroughly with distilled deionized water, dried with a clean lint-free towel, trimmed of inedible parts and damaged areas. They kept the peel for the apple and potato composites. Then they cut the fruit or vegetable into 1.25 cm pieces, quickly frozen in liquid nitrogen, and homogenized them with a food processor. This homogenized material was kept for twelve months. They found that fresh fruits and vegetables may be homogenized and stored frozen for up to 12 months with no loss of that natural methylated folate.

I thought that was so interesting, and it said a lot to me about how important processing is to the dense nutrients that our bodies are craving. It said a lot about the power or food over man-made vitamins, especially since my folate is coming in a powdered form of leafy greens and lemon peels. It said a lot about how despite our grandparents having the same mutations we have, this new world is a far different beast than we even realize. It is driving moms and dads, and kids to do crazy diets and take crazy weight loss supplements, or going to the extremes of gastric bypass because we don't know how to be a body. I used to be able to count the number of friends that had a gastric bypass done, and now I have lost count. How sad is it that this is our new normal? One woman told me once that she needed to gain weight to get the help she needed... surgically cutting ourselves up is just another Band-Aid. We have to get to the root causes.

I think we are trying to be the photo filter images we have created. God knows that I love a smooth face photo as much as the next person. We see the likes and we determine it to be love. What other habits have you created to get love/attention? People are being told they can have it all if they just give in, and yet when you look at a photoshopped picture of a gorgeous 40 year old grandma you don't always see the disclaimer that she has had $65,000 in work to look that way, plus a professional photographer and photoshop.

I think people that are buying into the "nextgen" supplements that are filled with the same synthetics as those multivitamins, are going to find that they are the same things to the body as the processed foods that we are trying to avoid. I think the gluten and polyunsaturated plant based meats are just as bad. High dose anything is not balanced. High dose exercise, high dose sugar, high dose supplements; none of this is what we want. Unnatural is not what we crave. Biohack to your heart's desire, but just know that if you don't tune in and have an awareness of what your body really needs, you will remain lacking. What you want is a balanced life, and a healthy body. That's the real happiness factor. We want balanced blood sugar, balanced cortisol, and balanced microbiome... balance. That is what I want to encourage everyone to seek in this adventure. We don't want any more diets, we just crave balance. Start with some simple meal prepping, and find a little balance.

As I created this entire knowledge dump that I wanted so badly to share, I wanted something balanced that was easy to duplicate. I also didn't want to take away from the feeling of happiness that I want you to associate with healthy foods. If tomorrow you couldn't ever eat a bit of cake, a juicy apple, a chocolate truffle, blueberry pie... the truth is that would be all you would think about.

I do want you to start with just one tough month of elimination, and ease in over four months to a sustainable lifestyle. You will learn to embrace the juicy micronutrients, and moments of simplicity for both body and soul. You will find that we are the creators of the generations to come, and diets are never going to be good energy. So it is time to stop. We are these Paleo 10 X bodies, yet forgetting the evolutionary foundational program. Put the fads down, and learn how to be in a body, and give yours what makes it work.

4

Elimination

Whoa, elimination. That's as close as you can get to a four letter word in my book. However I have been through it with all of my digestive issues, and all of my food allergies. I know just how important it is to be able to tag a food as an offender. Remember what I found when I gave up quinoa? When I thought about what I wanted this new book to be, I knew it had to create the possibility for change. Isn't that what brought you to it?

So how do you feel about this idea in this space in your life? Change. Fear. Excitement. Wellness. Nourishment. Probably a little of all of those things. What brought me to this is what started the full journey, which you have been invited to learn about. Once I had my daughter, I was 37, overweight and overwhelmed with everything. I had done a lot of changes in my lifetime due to so many different things. I let go of home grown to boxed foods when my mom went back to work. I let go of ingredients because I didn't quite know yet how to let go of the boxed foods. I tried traditional diets, fermented foods, the Whole30 multiple times. The truth for me is that it was always one step forward and two steps back.

I found after each of these changes that I still had asthma, I still had anxiety, I still had the bloat, the freezing histamine reactions after workouts, and there was only small moments that seemed to click. In 2019 from the previous Christmas to this Christmas I released twenty pounds. It was an energetic alignment that allowed me to open up and listen to what I truly wanted in this life. It was part loving myself and part letting my body guide my nutrition.

Years before when I was drinking this superfood shake daily before it was reformulated, it really worked for me. I started realizing that maybe it wasn't just the nutrition I had eliminated, but it was the easily absorbed nutrition and the energy I was adding in. Yet, I know that had I never gone Paleo when I was vegan I would not have realized what a huge problem so many foods were for my body. So a little nod of gratitude for the light on my trail.

You would think that having all of the food allergies I have, the severe IBD that I had suffered with, that I would have figured that nutrition thing out. But I didn't. I didn't for a long time. We are such pretty humans, but we are just not that smart. So don't see this process as a 30 day program because you are on a lifetime learning journey. As your body changes, your heart changes, your energy changes, your journey changes. Being open and aware to that will be the most relevant lifestyle change you can make, ever.

For this first month I recommend you call this your point A. You will have point Bs, and point Cs, and probably Point Zs and double AAs. It's not about rushing anything. You are the driver to be in charge of how long you continue, what foods to try to reintroduce, and who will decide what your lifestyle looks like going forward.

First we will ditch the glutinous grains, and dairy. When you eat gluten, when it reaches your intestines, tissue transglutaminase (tTG), an enzyme that is produced in your intestinal wall, breaks down the gluten into its protein building blocks, gliadin and glutenin. This can cause your gut cells to release zonulin, another protein that can break the tight junctions apart. We talk a lot in the nutrition community about the supplements and the bone broth to use to tighten up the junctions. Beyond telling you not to eat gluten, have you ever heard that it was a main cause due to the protein the gut releases rather than the protein you just ate? It is no wonder that with the high gluten levels in the wheat in the US we have come to a point of mass gluten-intolerance. That is because the two most powerful triggers to open this zonulin door is gluten, and your gut bacteria in the small intestine.

When people are not dealing with Celiac, but instead some sort of gluten intolerance, it is because we are breaking the junctions apart and leaking proteins into the bloodstream to be treated like an invader. Wheat, in particular, is a much harder product and has far higher levels of these proteins in the commercial wheat in the United States than in France or Italy. So you may be one of those people that has eaten pasta in Paris just fine, but can't stomach it when you get back home.

Gliadin is present in wheat as well as several other cereals within the grass family and can cross the intestinal barrier. The foods besides wheat that you have to really be careful of are barley and rye. Oats don't contain gluten but they do contain gliadin, and yet none of the currently known epitopes (which is the part of an antigen that is recognized by the immune system). None of those from wheat, barley, and rye occur in oats. So that makes it complicated for those trying to decide what is safe and what isn't. Oats are the most likely contaminated non-gluten food, so you have to make sure it's certified gluten-free if you are going to use them. Similar with quinoa some types have peptides which elicit a reaction similar to gluten in cell tests, or where cross contaminated. So any pseudo-grain can cause this reaction if the product has come into contact with gluten. Gluten-free certification matter because of this.

I also agree with eliminating corn, also known as maize, from your diet because corn in fact has similar proteins to gluten. It has been shown to act just like gliadin peptides in some people with gluten sensitivities. If you have gut problems, you should call yourself gluten sensitive because of its ability to cross over the gut barrier. I found that eliminating corn and corn-based products from my diet was the key to eliminating the daily barrage of my IBD symptoms in my twenties.

For this first thirty you are going to eliminate all of those, and then slowly reintroduce. I recommend starting with the non-gmo and certified gluten-free oat.

So what about the dairy? I have promoted in the past using an undenatured grass-fed whey protein if you are going to use it, however it is still not guaranteed to be free of casein. Casein inflames the gut just like gluten can. There was a study done with just 20 people with celiac that had been healing their guts for 2 years or more on a completely gluten-free diet. Ten were only in partial remission and still showed abnormal bowel biopsies, but negative gliadin and TG antibodies. Fifteen controls (15 people without Celiac Disease) were also tested. They used a rectal process and patches of cow's milk and casein which touched the mucosal wall. They were left for an hour. Fifteen hours later inflammatory responses were tested for. In 10 of the 20 CD patients the inflammatory response to casein or milk was similar to their reaction to a gluten rectal challenge. There was no or slight reaction in the controls. Casein has similarities to gliadin, high in proline and resistant to digestion, and has some similar amino acid sequences. If I have 4000 people in my nutrition groups, and 2,000 have gluten intolerance, 1,000 of us are going to react to dairy in exactly the same way that we react to gluten. So we just remove it to see how your gut does without it.

In my groups we generally have a high segment of vegans. Vegans are those that exclude all animal products, especially meat, seafood, poultry, eggs, and dairy products. This does not require consumption of whole foods or restrict fat or refined sugar. A lot of people do not follow a vegan lifestyle in the other areas of their life, like with abstaining from leather. These people sometimes feel more comfortable with the terminology plant based. I think as a whole most of the world is moving to a 90-10 plant based lifestyle. Also called Whole-food, Plant Based (WFPB) in this area you will eat lots of vegetables, fruits, legumes, seeds and nuts, with a lower fat consumption depending on if you are oil-free or not. There are those that are Raw Food, Vegan which means they have the same exclusions as vegans with the additional exclusion of all foods cooked at temperatures less than than 118°F. Many people that lean into veganism with juice cleanses will spend some time as raw vegans.

Vegetarians include some animal products, although there are many different flavors of vegetarianism. Lacto-vegetarians will exclude eggs, meat, seafood, and poultry and include pastured full-fat and fermented milk products. So if you fall in here you may try to reintroduce some pastured whey when you complete this initial informational portion of the program. Ovo-vegetarians will also exclude meat, seafood, poultry, and dairy products, and will include pastured eggs. Lacto-ovo vegetarians just exclude the meat, seafood, and poultry while including both the eggs and dairy products. There are other offshoots like Flexitarians that lean in and out of any one of these diets, or Pescatarians that usually eat like a Lacto-ovo Vegetarian, but with added Seafood. As you venture through this program, one of these may jump out to you as something you want to try as you reintroduce foods to your system.

In 2006, after reviewing data from 87 published studies, Susan E. Berkow, PhD, CNS Neal Barnard, MD reported in Nutrition Reviews that a vegan or vegetarian diet is highly effective for weight loss. This is why I am not surprised so many people get hooked on this diet. As well they found that vegetarian populations have lower rates of heart disease, high blood pressure, diabetes, and obesity. They determined in their studies that weight loss in vegetarians is not dependent on exercise and occurs at a rate of approximately 1 pound per week. The authors further stated that a vegan diet caused more calories to be burned after meals, in contrast to non-vegan diets which may cause fewer calories to be burned because food is being stored as fat.

Another study in the Journal of the American Medical Association reported that women with breast cancer who regularly consumed soy products had a 32% lower risk of breast cancer recurrence and a 29% decreased risk of death, compared with women who consumed little or no soy. I don't think they were looking at any of the modified, highly processed soy that has found its way into just about every boxed food in America, but organic and non-gmo soy that is minimally processed. An analysis of 14 studies, published in the American Journal of Clinical Nutrition has shown us that increased intake of this "good" soy resulted in a 26% reduction in prostate cancer risk. Because of concerns over the estrogenic nature of soy products, women with a history of breast cancer should discuss soy foods with their oncologists.

I highly recommend that you listen to, or purchase the hormone book written by Dr. Lindsey Berkson. She has delved so far into this area of research, being a survivor herself. She worked with hormones for a decade, and has very interesting perspectives that you don't usually find in conventional doctors. Just remember that overly processed, soy-based meat substitutes are often high in isolated soy proteins and other ingredients that may not be as healthy as less processed soy products (i.e., tofu, tempeh, and cold processed soy). This is why some low processed non-gmo & organic soy is allowed in my group that supports those doing my program, or looking for vegan or vegetarian support for their Whole30 program. However, if you have been eating a lot of bad soy products, exclude all soy from your 30 day diet (you won't die as I did strict W30 vegan for years without any soy) and give you gut a change to reevaluate it later.

This idea of getting started is the scariest part of this process, and so you've already overcome that by buying this book. My best tip is that as you jump in; create simple automated meals that you know you will enjoy.

What can you eat? You can choose any non-glutinous pseudo-grains, as well as properly prepared legumes if you desire, or go through thirty days completely grain-free. If you go completely grain-free you will need to make sure you get enough protein, perhaps through daily protein enriched green smoothie, or add some protein powder into chia pudding. I also love to make things different than a normal breakfast like a big roasted sweet potato bowl for breakfast.

We often host parties that we call Salad in the Jars where you get together with friends and each brings an item to add to your salads. This doesn't include your dressing or the greens. These lunches are so great because they are portable and you can just grab it and go once you add your greens and your little dressing container. I also have a meal prep group that focuses in on eating whole foods, made with healthy, non-gmo, gluten-free and non-irradiated spices. Spices are the flavor that will keep you coming back to real food.

Many of the popular challenge programs do not allow snacking, but if you have any sort of imbalance with your blood sugar levels you may just have to snack. Some people do just need the every three hours of a little protein and a little complex carbohydrate. It isn't for me to decide how your body works best. For me if I add in intermittent fasting, I have a lower risk of blood sugar imbalances. You can have gluten-free and dairy-free protein bars if you make them, fresh fruit, and as many veggies as you can eat, maybe even with some hummus. Maybe chew up a great digestive enzyme beforehand, or take some digestive bitters to help you actually digest the vegetables, and if you still can't, listen to your body. Find the foods that work for you.

You may also find yourself eating avocados as they go so far in helping sustain those sugar cravings as you are getting off sugar. I am not able to eat avocado, and so I make zucchini guacamole with algae oil to get those healthy mono-unsaturated fats in that I may be lacking otherwise. So many people come into these life changes with sugar cravings on overload. I recommend eliminating sugar, because it just feeds the bacteria you are trying to drive out. Sugar isn't all around a horrible thing, and a little is not the end of the world. Just understand that it is a trigger to a deeper drop when you have more than a couple grams at a time.

Then what's for dinner? I can always go for some soup, a healthy stir-fry or tonight we are having burrito bowls. If you can throw together the veggies you like and spice them up, you'll be fine. After dinner if you are still hungry I have two tricks. One is to try a nice warm herbal tea. I learned that little gem from Oprah at least a decade ago. Second is to have what we term at our house as second dinner. It's really just some wild blueberries with a little algae oil and non-dairy compliant milk on top. My daughter gets low blood sugar overnight and so when she gets hungry this is a way to help her body make it through the night well.

I always have great recipes in my group, and I have an online recipe portal where you can curate what you love to help you get through it. Just go to the Paleo Vegeo website and you can find links to both of those. Finding a few sauce ideas and dressing recipes is the easiest way to keep the flavor fun in your vegetable creations, and losing the feeling that you are somehow missing out.

As dieters we often don't think about how much nutrients impact our body. The biggest question I get from new clients is "what can I have for protein??" That question just expands because what people are really asking is about good sources of essential amino acids. Did you know that amino acids are the building blocks of making proteins or enzymes in the body? As well those aminos are the basis of the peptides that I talk about and work with as an energetic woo-woo dealer. You do not need to eat complete proteins as the media myths that have circulated for years have stated, and also note that all of your vegetables have some protein in them. A protein is nothing more than a chain of amino acids and 9 of the 20 some amino acids are considered essential because they have to come from the foods we eat. All of the other amino acids we can synthesize in our body. Your body is crazy amazing, isn't it?

Now the thing about proteins, as well as carbohydrates, as well as fats..... is that they fall into a larger category called macronutrients. Macronutrients provide those building blocks as well as the calories we need to keep the body going. This is what keeps you from being tired and hangry during your lifestyle changes. To explain the difference to people let me explain it in terms of the analogy of driving a car. In a car, you have gasoline and you have oil. To drive the human machine, you need.... similarly.... the gasoline and the oil. The gasoline, in this case, would be the macronutrient... which is the proteins, fats and carbohydrates found in food. So whenever you eat, you are ingesting proteins, fats and carbohydrates. That's why you need to eat.

Supplementation on top of that is not a major source of calories. They are not your macronutrients, and so you still need that rainbow of food to fuel your car. Supplementation provides micronutrients. You may be asking what is the micronutrient component of foods? It is the oil that makes the human body machinery run. It is involved in everything from our antioxidant function, to cell detoxification, and hormone regulation. Our micronutrients turn on and off genes. This ability of plant nutrients to turn on the good genes and turn off bad genes is something I think is super cool, and part of what really engaged me when I started this journey.

Plant nutrients are really, really important. Scientists believe there are over 25,000 plant nutrients. These are the micronutrients and include the minerals that are found in plants. If you aren't supplementing you aren't doing enough for your body. The soil that grows our fruits and vegetables has been depleted of nutrients, it is just a fact. Many wellness websites will tell you that oranges aren't just vitamin C; they're a huge array of complementary vitamins, minerals, and phytonutrients that work together synergistically to keep you healthy in ways that most studies say a vitamin C supplement just can't. I agree. That is why when I supplement I use mostly whole food supplements and they use the whole orange, not just the vitamin C. How often do you eat the peel of the orange? My amazing, genetically weird daughter eats the lemon peels. Since they are high in natural folate, who am I to stop her. Find your micronutrient Zen and you'll start to get your groove back.

5

Eat Your Superheroes

When I was just starting to write this book, I had three separate conversations in one day that had something to do with polyphenols. I think the universe was telling me to start sharing how essential this micronutrient is with my followers even though until that very moment it had just been pushed aside in the dream slot. Once you start to understand the need you will understand why I supplement for the polyphenol dietary gap eating whole foods every single day.

The first thing I realized as I increased my bad fats was that I also increased my inflammation. I had sore joints, and painful lymph glands. My entire lymphatic system became sluggish and felt almost as if it was clogged. I have stickier blood platelets, and I have to be very careful about watching my cholesterol. This is what you may have only read about after Bob Harper had his heart attack while doing CrossFit a few years ago. Our lymphatic system is essential to be able to clear oxidized cholesterol from our arterial walls. It is the balance beyond just dealing with waste products and toxins. The lymph system has a part in so many areas of our body. The mast cells and lymph nodes have a signaling process that happens every time I have a histamine release, and sometimes I don't care to have one. The lymphatic system creates those white blood cells to defend our body against disease. This amazing system even removes carbon dioxide and moves it back out of the body. I try to spend at least ten minutes every day on my vibration plate to help my lymphatic system do its job. Some people prefer to jump on a rebounder, but you know that some of us are more aligned with gravity and need to vibe and not jump. There are even lymphatic vessels in our brain microbiome, which may have to do with how this microbiota can cross the brain-blood-barrier. In fact small molecules of dietary polyphenols may cross the brain-blood-barrier as well, and it may have to do with how they work with our colonies of microbiome.

You know I talk a lot about the microbiome and how it impacts us so much; however did you know that polyphenols impact those microbiomes?? Polyphenols play a huge role in not only balancing the colonies of our gut but they also directly stimulate the vagus nerve to enhance digestion, pancreatic function, correct insulin response and are now being hugely studied as a cure for obesity. The vagus nerve indeed has a crucial role to play in our biliary system, and polyphenols are a part of what we need to help it along. Polyphenols fight yeast, candida, biofilm, and help shield our cells from oxidation. How does all of this happen?

First the good gut microbes feed off polyphenols. Most people that eat trend diets don't get a lot of polyphenols in their diet. The most they get may come in the form of low quality coffee products, which isn't going to give you what your body needs. In fact many low quality coffee beans are ripe with mold, and if you know me, you know my distaste for what mold does to the body. Just by adding in polyphenols not only are you supporting those good gut microbes, but they've been shown to help in the inhibition of carbohydrate digestion and glucose absorption in the intestine, stimulation of insulin secretion from the pancreatic β–cells, modulation of glucose release from the liver, activation of insulin receptors and glucose uptake in insulin-sensitive tissues, and modulation of intracellular signaling pathways and gene expression. (19) When you eat, your gastric system gets fired up if it's working properly, it is amazing. This is why when I was figuring out this new direction of eating, I decided that one day per week was going to be focused on eating only those healthy fruits and those fermentable vegetables that will make us feel much better and help us to get better results in the end. Write that down. One day a week focus in on eating just those healthy fruits and those fermentable vegetables. See how that feels and listen to your awareness.

Part of what our gastric system does that is essential to our body is activating our vagal receptors with a sort of "dosing" from the reactions that are taking place due to your happy little colony of microbiota. So not only are you using the nutrients more effectively, but if you eat well that tells your body what is going on with the meal and you stop being hungry all of the time. It's not just the healthy fats that help you to be satiated; it's that well running gastric machine.

There are chemical vagal responses triggered on these same receptors, which is why when you eat artificial sweeteners your response is to stay hungry. Interesting enough is that you can also stimulate your vagus nerve through light or via compression of the mucosa in your gut. Those polyphenols in the skins of fruits and vegetables, grains and seeds are there for us, and thanks to nature being in sync with our physical body. The secret is to find the ones that you can digest well, and thus make your body run more efficiently. My green tea latte and blueberries in the mid-morning to early afternoon are fantastic. Similarly I love black cumin oil, pomegranates, celery juice and basil. So many good polyphenols out there to help the vagus thrive.

This vagus nerve is the longest cranial nerve, and up to 90% of the vagus nerve fibers are sensory nerves that are communicating with the brain. Stimulating vagal afferent fibers in our gut influences brain systems in the brain stem that play crucial roles in major psychiatric conditions, such as mood and anxiety disorders. And in fact those hormones and peptides that the enteric nervous system, or second brain, releases to cross the blood-brain-barrier, act synergistically with the vagus nerve. This has opened up an entirely new area of treatment between nutrition and psychiatric, inflammatory and neurological conditions.

I have talked before in classes about peptides. I like to think of a peptide by thinking about rays of sunshine. The Sun shines down and touches many things, yet it does only one thing. Shine. Peptides are really just short little pieces of proteins, that are not dangerous, just amino acids that are made up of the same elements that make up our beings. The pattern of the "beads on the string" is what makes peptides bioactive. Think again about the sunshine. How different is a sunset out in the desert and a sunset over the ocean?

Each unique pattern of these "beaded strings" can be recognized by our immune system, but the origin of the peptide is not encoded in the sequence of amino acids or as we are calling them, beads. A peptide from a cancer cell and from a chicken sandwich can be exactly the same pattern.

When this happens, the immune system can get confused and stop attacking the cancer. When a unique peptide is recognized in the digestive tract, the immune system is trained to shut down responses toward the food peptides. So the peptide message to the cancer cell may be because another peptide had the same pattern and thus told it to activate. Where there are proteins there are peptides. Every whole food, every bacteria and living organism is full of peptides that can be evaluated by our immune system. And this all seems to be centralized to that digestive system, and the little colony of bacteria that reside within it. And as I have said we carry the microbiota not just in our gut, but on our skin.

Everything that is going on in your life right now has to do with peptides. How much of any one particular peptide that you have in your system right now and how it's impacting you comes down to all that you are. Those people we are sitting here with right now, the measurable thoughts we are having, what you had for lunch today, and the lingering essential oil aromas or chemical toxins right here in this very room. But most importantly is how that makes you feel. And how many emotions do we have throughout the day. Especially if you consider all of the stimulation in our lives from video games, social media, relationships, school, sugar, processed foods, and more.

So the kicker, energy beings is this: How much of a particular peptide you have available and active in your body is directly impacted by, among other things, by your emotional experiences. Negative activities, negative foods, negative thinking is like a brick wall preventing you from manifesting, from receiving because it becomes the driver for your being. There are so many things that come together to create positive thinking or negative thinking. You learn to control that, and you learn to receive. We learn that when we drink a cup of freshly pressed greens or take in encapsulated foods or eat healthy non-gmo foods that it shares the enzymes to break down the peptides to activate all of the good we desire in our life. As a cellular being we are electricity and pathways for chemical reactions. Both good and bad.

So as a vast and expansive energy being, this wandering nerve of electricity within us touches our gut, our heart, our brain and just about every organ you can think of in between. There is a hormone called CCK, which is often found in the small intestines. This is what tells you that you've eaten enough. So eating well can trigger that entire process and then it suddenly connects to why when I get my daily micronutrients I am often just not hungry afterwards. That is one of those second brain connections.

For those of you that have done any sort of fasting or Bulletproof coffee to start your day, it helps explain why you don't want to eat until midafternoon. It's the best part of intermittent fasting in my opinion. Every morning I enjoy a tea made with turmeric (which I am going to talk more about later), ginger, algae oil, sometimes a little Brain Octane oil, water and sometimes a sprinkling of either coconut cream or homemade hemp milk. Healthy fatty acids trigger the CCK just like healthy foods. It also causes the release of digestive enzymes and bile from the pancreas and gallbladder, and that makes digesting those fats easier. Researchers are looking at the different levels of CCK in very obese people, compared to less obese and slimmer individuals. So far the findings are linking having less CCK can be associated with obesity. Like MTHFR, this is a genetic variant that they are just learning about. Welcome to what may be the genetic revolution.

Similar research I have looked into shows our cannabinoid pathway can also regulate like a healthy fat or healthy polyphenol. Animal studies showed that rats given CBD ate much less food than the control group, as CBD has been shown to increase leptin levels. For a few years leptin has been the much talked about "starvation hormone". Now we are finally learning why these select items work, and learning which are considered the best.

When we eat polyphenols our microbiome release these neuroactive mediators to do more than just tell us we're satiated, and more than just release those digestive juices. These polyphenols do some amazing things to the vagus nerve. Alternatively when we eat cow's milk and wheat gluten there is also a release that can say, "Hey... this is making us not feel well" and can trigger mast cell histamine reactions. I read a study using apples, and what the researchers saw was that these extracts from the immature fruit of the apple (Rosaceae, Malus sp.), were able to inhibit histamine release from mast cells. It was the polyphenols at work and the reason why I use a lot of nettle and quercetin when I am dealing with mast cell chaos. This is also a reason why I am so sure that if you ditch the dairy and gluten for some time, and start eating more of what I call high vibrational foods, you'll start to see some changes in how you feel. However just getting rid of the inflammatory foods when we have an internal mess isn't going to fix the problem. It can take decades to fully heal your gut from the decades of damage you have done through the simple love of eating a gloriously comforting piece of bread.

So why does it matter if we take a bunch of powdered whole foods into our diet? For me it's about eating more dense nutrition that remains whole. I know there is no way I can eat all of these foods in one day in any other way. I once looked at the dietary protocol for MS and couldn't imagine eating three pounds of produce a day. I don't have a large enough fridge, I won't eat them all, and some of them I won't digest any other way. For me it was that getting all of those whole foods in encapsulated compounds that have all of the synergy like retaining the methylfolate in the greens. I read up on those same compounds used orally or via intravenous forms of delivery in the clinical models, and the difference it created. I follow the science and the collected data, and this is what has been found to have the greatest ability to make it through the digestion and metabolism to impact the biological effects from the polyphenols that we desire.

I do read a lot of clinical research, because I am a geek, and what I have found is that just eating foods rich in polyphenols doesn't cut it. You need to know that before you get started with these changes. They are currently working on some neurotherapeutic application polyphenols for Alzheimer's Disease because of the way that these antioxidants shield nerve cells in the brain, but I think that's going to take some time. In the meantime it's really pretty amazing how many ways these micronutrients impact quality of life, but you have to get them into your diet first. Your vagus nerve and your microbiome cannot do what we desire without the proper nutrition. Just eating the traditional high saturated fat, latest trend diet, unless it is for medical purposes, isn't going to be as healing as you crave. Even those on medical ketogenic diets know that "a ketogenic diet should consist of whole foods that are organic, high in fiber, and sourced from one's local environment." The Charlie Foundation has been helping people for over twenty years to lower seizures using a whole food, high fiber ketogenic dietary plan. Remember how I said we are out gut, and our gut is us?

There are so many studies out there on the vagus nerve, and most of those that I have read recently are focused on stimulation. Vagus nerve stimulation has been approved in epilepsy and treatment resistant depression, and that is hopefully just the beginning. Because of these studies and other migraine studies suggesting vagus nerve stimulation could reduce migraines (common in ME/CFS and FM) and also pain, even more studies are being done. (Hooray!) Generally in medical practice vagus nerve stimulation is done through surgery and implants. The catch is the cost. VGS, as it is called, is approved for epilepsy but not for pain.

This is another little bit of information from my intuitive domino tracking being, and I believe it all starts at birth with an infection since several infections can be transmitted from mother to child. So there is more than just genetics or epigenetics at play. This has been called the Vagus Nerve Infection Hypothesis (VNIH). And it is also why our gut health is so important. Consider what is happening if the bacteria in our gut is constantly chatting it up with our vagus nerve. The medical belief is that these cells cause immune activation, and that vagus nerve stimulation could stop that continued cycle.

We can have an infection in our body that is not showing up in our blood tests, we know this and we read it all of the time. Ever read about false negatives? A friend was recently tested negative to having H. Pylori, however the high levels of carbon dioxide in her body was telling quite the opposite story. If we go back to those infections that started all of this, and the biofilm they protect themselves with, these same polyphenols can disrupt the metabolism and structural components of these cells. I've seen amazing studies taking place in regards to candida biofilm. I also recently had eaten some of the bad romaine when I had just replanted my urban indoor garden. I didn't really feel that sick, and so I didn't think much of it until I got E-coli infused UTI. Did you know that the most common cause of UTI's is E-coli bacteria?

If we look at a familiar story, we can talk about the keto rash that I thought I had when I started struggling in the summer. When people start eating high fat diets there are a number of reactions that are taking place that can cause this miserable reaction. The keto rash means your lymph system may be sluggish. I knew this to be true from the swollen lymph glands I was dealing with. You are also dumping out toxins and histamine from your fat cells and your already overworked liver is struggling to keep up. You also could likely have some biofilm resistance that you are dealing with, and your skin doesn't like the chemicals your body is releasing. And finally, of course, you need to eat more carbs because your body needs the fiber and micronutrients. For those that this doesn't impact you may feel lucky; however you are still doing a disservice to your gut if you aren't eating enough fiber and polyphenols.

We now know you need a lot of polyphenols, at least 1,000 mg per day. That's a lot. And these are the key defense systems for plants to fight off microbial invaders, which is why they work for us. As a population we have 10 times more microbes in our gut than anywhere else in our body, there are also around 1,000 types of microbes on our skin. So doesn't it make sense for us to also have these complex defensive weapons available for our body by consuming enough of them? You probably take or eat some sort of probiotic, or probiotic rich foods, right? Unlike probiotics, polyphenols are more robust in their ability to reach the lower intestine. However, just like probiotics you have to take enough polyphenols, and the right polyphenols, in order to reach that destination and have a therapeutic effect in the gut. So just remember that not any old polyphenol will do just like not any old probiotic will do. Many species that you get in your daily probiotic are high histamine producing, and so you may actually want to focus in on the prebiotics instead for this first month. You get that from the fiber and resistant starches you are eating.

So how would you like to join me and start to change your body? I get 600 mg of polyphenols daily via whole micronutrients. Dave Asprey talks all the time about how much rosemary he eats, and I'm like, Dave... it would take 38 tsps. of rosemary to get this much polyphenols in my diet. I love rosemary, but there is no current possibility that I would eat that much in a day. Approximately 5% of the dry weight of rosemary leaves is comprised of the phenolic diterpenes, and so maybe the answer we will find is in using rosemary oil. For now though, I will take my route of encapsulated foods. Aren't we working towards having the most expensive urine on the planet? Just kidding, as I am sure he wins in that category. I would love to know if he is super biohacking his rosemary, and the various types of high polyphenol supplementation he takes daily.

There are lots of polyphenol rich foods we can eat, however drinking one of my favorite cups of matcha green tea will only get you 1 gram of polyphenols. I don't know anyone that wants to, or would feel good drinking 10 cups of matcha per day. I am a fast caffeine metabolizer, but not that fast. A handful of cloves will get you another gram of polyphenols, and yet I am not going to eat even a handful. If you wanted to make a chia smoothie, you could definitely soak them to toss in the blender tomorrow. I know several people that swear by this. Berries, apples, peaches, apricots, pears, green grapes and sweet cherries like they grow in the Rainier Valley are also very rich in polyphenols. They are a great way in the summer to get some extra boosts, and really important since they have this ability to protect the skin from the adverse effects of UV radiation, including the risk of skin cancers. (10) So nature is pretty smart to make that a benefit in a summertime fruit. Most of the polyphenols are found in the seeds of the berries, and in the peels of citrus fruits. This is why those rich omegas in seeds are being studied for their skin protective benefits.

The polyphenols in tea, apples and onions only have to make it past the stomach and into the small intestine to convert to quercetin and epicatechins, two important polyphenol flavanols. I love eating a rich, juicy gala apple with some hummus or a handful of olives. Have you ever eaten brownie hummus? It is one of those items I consider to be the nectar of the Gods. Flavonoids are the most common polyphenol group found in our diet today. They are the part of the plant that attracts the pollinator honey bee, fights off environmental stress and regulates cell growth. In Traditional Chinese Medicine they are connected to managing blood sugar levels, balancing blood pressure and protecting the skin from UV radiation. The flavonoids are very anti-inflammatory in nature.

Two of my favorite vegetables in this category are celery and parsley. I wasn't into celery as a juice until Anthony Williams, the Medical Medium, came into my radius. Knowing that compassion is the key to vagal tone, and that the Spirit that he works with is the word, Compassion; for me it seems to be another synchronicity I needed to absorb into my journey. They say that these two vegetables, juiced, are the secret key to stop storing so much bad fats in our belly. As I started creating a rich change in my style of vegan living, I added in at least sixteen ounces a day of cold pressed greens, celery included. Watching as my belly deflated was a sure sign that the micronutrients were working. Flavonoids encourage our body to use those fats, rather than store fat, because of the detoxifying qualities of their polyphenol bodies.

For men parsley can boost your testosterone levels, and for women it can lower our risk of ovarian cancer. (11) The secret is in the apigenin, which researchers at Texas Tech University found to be a promising testosterone booster. What intrigued me about that research was the benefit to increasing bone density, liver function, and reducing the risk of neurodegenerative diseases. The neuronal loss in different neurodegenerative diseases like Multiple Sclerosis and ALS are being researched because there is a debate on whether it is the cause, or the inflammatory reaction. Apigenin, again for women, inhibits the self-renewal capacity of human ovarian cancer SKOV3-derived sphere-forming cells research discovered. (12) Most of the apigenin is found in the celery leaves, as well as parsley. I also love that it is found in cilantro because my favorite pressed juice contains both celery and cilantro. I think it's important to note that these specific flavonoids occur predominantly in their leaves.

Can you guess my favorite go to for extra polyphenols through the afternoon is? I am going to encourage you to eat what my husband calls dirt, otherwise known as dark chocolate (of course it's dark chocolate not diarylicious chocolate). As I said when I get tired I crave copper. Dark chocolate is not just a rich source of polyphenols, but because of that it is a rich prebiotic for some pretty important gut microbes. If you look at the research for dark chocolate you'll find that it's believed to stop the root cause for persistent cough. It helps with those mood regulating chemicals, which also come from the gut. It triggers that "starvation hormone" we started talking about before, and so it will help you feel fuller. Most importantly a recent study reported that treatment with dark chocolate prevents the inflammation of the vagus nerve. (6) Since the study's now links vagal tone to inflammation and autoimmunity (13), of course it's something we all need to take a deeper look into.

In the meantime, just enjoy these rich foods, and know you are doing something helpful for your body. I am playing around with the idea of doing an elimination of even the dark chocolate again, back to the copper thing. I'll keep you informed on social media if I do, and how that works out as I have this working amnesia to any results when chocolate is eliminated from my diet. When I stopped eating dark chocolate for my Facebook challenge group, and increased those PUFA's I may have ramped up my inflammation in the vagus nerve. Can I link it to the lack of dark chocolate, who is to say. It only took four weeks for my body to go haywire and start feeling these effects. Of course I am not on medication, and so if I were it may have taken longer.

6

Stimulate Your Body

Vagus nerve inflammation is probably not something you may have ever even heard about before reading that last chapter. You may have never even heard of the vagus nerve at all. So now you know the vagus nerve is supposed to be the one to keep inflammation in check in our bodies, and for those of us with an autoimmune disorder we know all about inflammation. Medications for autoimmune diseases are also meant to lower the inflammation and bring some Zen to the overactive immune response. There are so many known and unknown items, however, that can cause the vagus nerve to be and do just the opposite of what we want it to.

So many people have their gallbladders out each year. In my old neighborhood I could throw a rock and hit a house where someone had theirs taken out, so I know a lot of those people. In fact, one of my best friends had her gallbladder out, and then still continued to have even more trouble than she started with. For all of the years we had known each other she suffered from an 'autoimmune' disorder, as well as severe acid reflux. If I had known years ago what I know now about vagus nerve dysfunction, I think it could have changed her outcome.

The gallbladder depends on the vagus nerve, and as such when it's dysfunctional your gallbladder will not function properly. For many of us it feels initially just like a little acid reflux. Unlike acid reflux, gallbladder pain isn't as easily pushed aside. It also is a denser pain, for me anyway. My daughter was diagnosed at four months with acid reflux or extreme colic nighttime screamer, and they started her on an acid reflux medication. Long term use of these drugs can lead to an excess of gastrin in the blood. That is part of the concern with using it daily over long periods of time. My daughter was on them for a few months, and then I took her off because it didn't seem to be the cause, or give the effect we desired. I could already see that when she wouldn't breastfeed, and we put her on Dr. Sears' goat milk formula, she was fine. When they pulled her off the goat milk and put her on expensive chemically laden formulas, she would scream. It was a direct reaction and they just were not connecting the dots. The truth about colic is that it can result from vagal nerve irritation more often than not. This is why those stomach massages work wonders by increasing vagal tone. They have found that infants often have colic as a symptom of anxiety and irritability of the central nervous system. Where do they get that anxiety? Generations and generations of family that has passed it along to them. Also new moms, have you ever felt a little anxiety about your newborn or your ability to care for them? Enough said.

Certain fibers of our vagus nerve within our stomach cells release a peptide that stimulates the release of gastrin. Remember those CCK hormones we talked about and the peptide emotional connection? Circulating gastrin indirectly works on the stomach enterochromaffin-like (ECL) cell CCK receptors. Because of this, histamine stimulates what is called parietal cell acid secretion, which is the hydrochloric acid, by binding to the parietal cells basolateral histamine 2 receptor. H2-receptor antagonists like these cause a 70–90% decrease in gastric acid production. H2 medications is what they give you for acid reflux, or out of control mast cells. Thankfully I am allergic to these medicines, and have to rely on natural alternatives.

These antagonists inhibit the digestion of protein in our stomach, and these undigested protein fragments can trigger an immune response or generate allergic responses. I spy a circle of problems right there. They are finally starting to look at the role these drugs can play in the development of childhood allergies. As well H2 receptors are not just in the stomach cells. These receptors are also located on cells in the heart, uterus, and the smooth muscles of the blood vessel wall that provides structural integrity, as well as regulating the vessel diameter by contracting and relaxing. Within certain autoimmune phenomenon there is destruction of these vascular smooth muscle cells, although they have no idea why. This is also something seen in women that have hypertension and polycystic ovarian syndrome. I just about threw up when I saw that they were doing research into unilateral or bilateral vagotomy for women with PCOS, especially when vagus nerve stimulation could be part of the answer. Gag reflex for me is an energetic bullshit call. Instead of enhancing our body's proper functionality, our processing system goes for cutting things out, like the gallbladder, rather than getting to the source.

When my pain wasn't just stomach pain, but also acid reflux symptoms, pain between my shoulders and finally a major ammonia dump, I knew I wasn't having heartburn. I dealt with severe IBD when I was younger, and this wasn't the same sort of problem. Ammonia dumping is often seen in high level athletes when the nervous system is overloaded, and it often shows up in the liver. As I have said, our liver requires vagal stimulation for the production and release of bile into the gallbladder. Ammonia levels in the blood rise when the liver is not able to convert ammonia to urea. One day after I started having these stomach pains I went roller skating with my daughter. When I came out to the car my shirt smelled like I had poured permanent waving solution all over it. At least as a licensed cosmetologist that is what it smelled like to me. My body was obviously having problems detoxing which caused the ammonia to come out through the skin, but also it was also a sign of what was impacting my gallbladder. I started to question if I actually could have created gallstones.

Yes, I knew I wasn't having a heart attack, before you stroll down that lane. Once I was aware of the ammonia, it was a big clue to what was going on. Believe me when I say that the pain in my biceps that night and the muscle weakness was awful. I actually took a steroidal medication because I was in that much pain. I followed that up with a big flushing niacin. That domino forced me to start directing my holistic approach to a pretty annoyed gallbladder. Something to consider is that when people usually have severe gallbladder pain they end up in the ER where they get their gallbladder removed. If it's related to the vagus nerve, or when the vagus nerve is cut during the operation, the problem just gets worse. These types of surgeries are often a cause of gastroparesis, which is damage to the vagus nerve causing digestive issues in the stomach.

Have you ever heard a doctor refer to 4F? This is their way of referring to your family history, gender, weight and being over forty. Family. Female. Fat Forty. They aren't concerned with your vagus nerve when they see you as just being 4F.

They now have a term called aging-related vagal tone, and in digestive issues they are calling it aging-related vagal withdrawal and they are looking at it for diverticular diseases. That is how integrated this nerve is to our bodily functions. (7) I was vegan so it really still made no sense why I would have gallstones when they occur after cholesterol and other substances found in bile form stones. They don't know why, but risk of symptomatic gallstone disease can be higher in women who are plant-based. My belief is that my body adjusted itself to low amounts of fat on my allergy-friendly, low fat, vegan diet and my gallbladder was not producing the amount of bile it needed to. Also I wasn't eating the foods that would help my gallbladder relax and do its job.

My family genetics, of course, leave me with higher than usual calcification; as well I have the increased cholesterol in my system when I ramped up my vegan fatty choices. Either of these could have sparked the problem. I was doing one heck of job of eating high amounts of cruciferous veggies, and I have the CBS mutation which can leave me with high levels of ammonia anyway. I have a defective homocysteine metabolism, and here I was eating more foods that did not agree with my mutation and more foods that did not help anything in my methylation pathway. I didn't realize how far off I was with my dietary choices until I was doing my own Dr. Google research that and had that a-ha moment that I needed to address the CBS mutation first, and I wasn't. The fact that my BH4 (co-factor for converting nitrogen to nitric oxide) has a direct correlation to my gallbladder since it restores gastric emptying, was that moment. Thank you MTHFR mutation for that little bit of added gastric assistance. (Sarcasm)

Things that can provoke high ammonia for those with my mutation are higher doses of essential fatty acid. Check! And I needed to be careful with sulfur because of its role in CBS upregulation. So lower garlic, broccoli, onions (I have onion soup EVERY Sunday in the winter), milk thistle, along with the bag of cruciferous vegetables I was eating every day. I was personally lowering my BH4 levels out of purely just not being aware. I think genetic knowledge is the best thing we can do for ourselves, and I wish it was a part of the first years of our life. Instead it is not until we are feeling down and out that we start to think about it and we go out and pay for it ourselves. I think for those with the CBS mutation, or even those with the MTHFR mutation and others, there is a nutrient power that we need to be aware of in our diet. If you have brain fog, it may need to be written out on your fridge because otherwise you will NEVER remember it.

Sulfur is great in an herb like parsley or spirulina and doesn't seem to cause the same problems as eating a herd of cruciferous vegetables. Guess who wasn't using those lovely herbs? By the way, I love herbs. They are magical and high in vibrations. I love adding a magical blue into my cold pressed green juice. With all of the knowledge you now know about parsley, I'm guessing it is going on your shopping list. I also know why tiny amounts of spirulina and cracked chlorella in my diet years ago were such a great thing, and large amounts are not. I always talk about personal nutritional truth, and finding your personal nutritional truth. Although many people would say that a high fat diet is the key, never forget that a huge shift in your diet shouldn't be started without understanding your genetics, your current system functionality, and what impact your current diet could have on the outcome of change.

At this point what I really needed to be doing for my body was increasing my vitamin C, and drinking my parsley juice. As well to get rid of the ammonia I increased my chlorophyll, zeolite spray, calcium bentonite clay and activated charcoal. Take all of those away from any medications or supplementation you are using since they are binders. You can also add some yucca root into your diet when you eat protein. I started thinking about how all of those amino acids impact everything. Just a little methionine is a good thing, too much can be bad. Just a little ammonia is a good thing, too much can be bad.

When we have too much protein (too much amino acids) our body tries to break down amino acids for energy. Then the amine group is removed from the amino acid and converted to ammonia. In the body what breaks down the amino acids is called deamination, and it mostly takes place in our liver. And where does bile get started? Our gallbladder holds bile produced in the liver until it is needed. Another little secret we probably needed to know.

I was still dealing with a pain that may or may not be a gallstone related to all of this. If it was a stone, passing from the gallbladder into the small intestine or maybe even becoming stuck in the biliary duct could be what was causing this pain. I started drinking a concoction of apple cider vinegar, artichokes, beets, blueberries, calcium, phyllanthus niruri, cinnamon, dandelions, hibiscus, honey and yes a little of the sulfur items and so I was not taking it three times a day like they suggested. Beets have been wonderful because they relax things by softening the bile duct so that if there is a gallstone, it can get through. I now drink beet juice whenever I am going to be eating those high sulfur foods. This concoction helped pretty quickly to relax the pain. However, what made the biggest difference was going into my office, shutting the door and doing a little yoga, Reiki and meditation. Sometimes connecting to that Zen is what we need, because it's what our vagus nerve needs.

Sometimes I think the vagus nerve is actually the physical embodiment of our energetic being. What I find the greatest about this research into the vagus nerve is that we're finding that when you are compassionate, you have a higher vagal tone. Mudras can help balance our vagus nerve, especially in the case where gastrointestinal bloating and indigestion that may be caused by overstimulation of the vagus nerve. There has to be a balance in all things, and it doesn't always mean what we think. The compassion research was led by Dacher Keltner at the University of California at Berkeley. I know that meditation was very helpful and opened me up to some possibilities that I didn't think of before to start healing this issue from the inside, while my vagal tone was doing its part from the real inside. Mindset and mudras were hitting at my door and I was really in need of it. Funny how all of this nutrition knowledge was lighting up the foundation for the work I needed to do in the energy field. This didn't just spark me to write this book, it sparked me to create an energetic awakened transcendence. So that is pretty powerful and speaks to the mind-body-soul connection.

I also say balance because we can get too much of a good thing. Over stimulation in the vagus nerve can be associated with anxiety, panic attacks, PTSD, insomnia, tinnitus, and irritable bowels. Underactive symptoms can be that slow gastric emptying, depression, and then again that anxiety, difficulty or discomfort when swallowing, and chronic inflammation. The reason why when having the gallbladder taken out, or having your stomach stapled they need to start doing education about the damage that will happen to the vagus nerve. With under stimulation and low gastric secretion, you can be missing the factor needed to absorb nutrients especially that much needed vitamin B12, and minerals. How many people end up in the ER post gastric surgery because they are in a state of seriously deficient micronutrients?

If you have an autoimmune disorder have you ever heard of pernicious anemia? You may know that there are underlying factors that may make your body more likely to have a deficiency in B12; however pernicious anemia is an autoimmune disease that created an inability to absorb your B12 in food. I know a lot of people don't realize they need to supplement with B12, or what type they should look into. Sometimes B12 deficiency can be corrected by just replacing or increasing bile, and sometimes it is more than that. This is where working with a great Functional practitioner can be helpful to figure out what to use for targeted supplementation, and what form. There are so many types of B-vitamin supplements out there on the market, and you need to know which one is right for you. We need that B12 for our nervous system, and our vagus nerve stimulates what is needed to absorb it. One serious side effect you never hear about in a vagotomy, or when your vagus nerve has been cut during surgery is a vitamin B12 deficiency. Now you know.

You also may not know this, but mindful meditation has been proven to also increase our vagal tone, and it can be measured by heart rate variability. So perhaps when I slowed down for meditation and energy work I was doing far more for my gallbladder pain than I realized. The more I have learned about the vagus nerve and the dysfunctions related to it, the more I know I have to target a Zen life if I want a long, healthy life. I have even created a deck of oracle cards to open up to mindful possibilities (called Mindset Unicorn cards) because I felt that having a push towards that daily vagal tone was so important to our health. Opening yourself up to mindful possibilities every day is something that can change the way you feel, and live.

If we move a little further in the questioning realm, if there is a group of compounds that have been found to help modulate this system, why aren't they being talked about?

Research has already shown anti-inflammatory effects with both polyphenols and another favorite of mine, essential oils. Essential oils and aromatherapy can help us in so many ways that we don't even understand yet. I do know that when I put the right aroma into my diffuser, the Zen opens up wide. This is the very reason why I wrote my book, 'Exploring Aromatherapy'. People have no idea of the safety, essential oils are everywhere, and they have uses beyond what is being talked about in the subtle body. It is that very inner being (or I could say outer since the inner energy can expand throughout the universe) having a release of olfactory emotions.

So would you be surprised if I told you that they found with increased polyphenols in our diet there is an increase in neuron birth in the two areas of the brain where neurogenesis (the growth and development of nervous tissue) is produced, the olfactory bulb and the hippocampus. (8) The hypothalamus is the message station for transmitting aroma messages to other areas of the brain. Oxytocin, the cuddle or love hormone is produced primarily in the hypothalamus. One of the mutated kids in our family was recently prescribed Oxytocin after having a genetic test to find the best medication for her anxiety. Practices are catching up slowly to the research and tools available.

If compassion is the most Important factor for our vagal tone, then this is where the motherlode lives. (9) Is this new knowledge how we will one day stop some of the damage to our brains, and our memories? I don't know, but as a

Certified Aromatherapist, Energy Facilitator and Nutritional Coach, I do know that it's exciting to see the direction all of this research is heading.

Have you ever met someone that suddenly had an autoimmune disease that defied diagnosis? It's not as uncommon as I would have thought. There are so many things that can trigger this autoimmune response in our system. I personally think we should start diagnosing ourselves as having inflammatory reflex with fetal related infections. My ADHD guide wants to bring you back to that space where I was just several pages ago. I think we should all get our genetic testing done to understand what is happening in our bodies, and I believe that struggling wellness issues are a combination of all of these things, but can be helped and many parts of the autoimmunity can be healed. My first practical advice, eat those polyphenols, and do a little something meditative now and again. Energy Work isn't just needed. Built as receptors we require it for optimal living.

Now of course if I am going to talk about stimulating our body, I have to talk about stimulating your lymphatic system. It is amazing that so many of the ways we can stimulate our vagus nerve will also stimulate your lymphatic system. Doing yoga, meditation, whole body vibrations, deep breathing and even drinking polyphenol-rich teas can all stimulate your lymphatic system. Are you surprised to learn that dandelions contain major polyphenols?

Milk thistle is also another wonderful nutrient that you can add to your dandelion tea to help aid your liver in its daily duties. Silymarin is a flavonoid concentrate of milk thistle, and it's very protective in regards to the liver. Since I have found so many of my own family members have to support their livers due to genetic storage issues, I have started being more aware of how much my little liver does for me every day. If you are going to start stimulating your body, you better work on stimulating your liver. Our next area of reset will need every bit of support your liver can get.

7

Heavy Metal Nation

You're hip, you're Zen and you still have an autoimmune disorder. How fracked up does that seem? There is more to your puzzle than just eating a handful of wild blueberries before yoga. Many autoimmune disorders have a direct connection to bacterial endotoxins. Endotoxins are toxins that are present inside of a bacterial cell. Once the cell disintegrates, the toxins are released. The two biggest contributors to our chronic disease are endotoxemia and immune hypersensitivity. There is very little known about how the vagus nerve modulates systemic inflammatory responses to endotoxins. One reason I have wanted to get an infrared sauna for so long is not just because of the support of detoxification, removing ammonia, and because it can be very supportive in clearing out all those endotoxins in the body.

I have a smaller 1970's house, and so trying to find room for an office, energy table, whole body vibration plate, treadmill, workout room... and you have to have room to sleep, eat and cook; so I have no room for an infrared sauna. However, I found a low emf sauna blanket that was created in part by Dr. Raleigh Duncan, Founder of Clearlight Saunas. I have the emf reading video on my YouTube channel. This blanket is an amazing biohacking tool that costs far less than a high quality sauna costs, and you can pack it up and take it with you when you are traveling on road trips. I find that many hotel rooms are full of toxins and mold, and by the time I get back from being on the road for several weeks my system is a wreck. Any tools I can use to support my body, if it is great and affordable I will share them.

There is a term called mercury-induced autoimmunity. Lipopolysaccharide (LPS) is the major component of the outer membrane and is another name for endotoxins. Mercury toxicity will make you more susceptible to LPS damage. I recently saw a study where they showed that when mercury attaches to the thiol protein in the heart muscle receptors (which is the proteins that regulate and/or modulate the physiology of heart functions) and in the acetylcholine (the neurotransmitter released by the vagus nerve), the heart muscle cannot receive the vagus nerve electrical impulse for contraction. Sounds pretty scary, right? I really think so because of the hole in my lower tricuspid valve of my heart that I have had since birth.

Many, many years ago I started a crusade for glutathione. In fact, I think those are some of my most popular blog posts. Glutathione maintains our defense system, and is the mother of all antioxidants. These endotoxins can cause a significant glutathione reduction, which impacts your detoxification in the body. This information is very relevant to the autism community since the similarities between autism and other autoimmune diseases suggest that autoimmunity may be a critical factor in the cause of autism. (14)

What triggers or turns on the genes of an autoimmune disorder that has been lying dormant in the body? Since World War II there has been a dramatic increase in the environmental toxins, and these could be a part of what triggers what the NIH calls a pandemic of more than 80 autoimmune disorders. A pandemic? Yes, the NIH is now calling the rise of autoimmune disorders a pandemic. The NIH says the environmental factors that trigger autoimmune disorders can include chemical toxicants, heavy metals, viruses, bacteria, emotional stress, and drugs. (15)

Smoking runs rampant in my family tree, and it's a known risk for RA. I have several family members with rheumatoid arthritis (RA) and one with psoriasis as well. She doesn't smoke, but her mother did. I can remember when I was a teen hanging out downstairs with my Aunt when we were visiting Pennsylvania, as she smoked one cigarette after another.

I also have another family member that was diagnosed with Hepatitis C. Many Hep C patients develop additional inflammatory disorders related to autoimmunity. They can also be misdiagnosed due to an underlying genetic mutation that causes hemochromatosis, which then causes liver damage. With a parent and two siblings dealing minimally with this genetic mutation, I find it interesting that it's also an unknown variant.

What about silicone implants? They may be one of the biggest autoimmune triggers as they have been connected to lupus, RA, and many other autoimmune illnesses. So genetics and environment go hand in hand in turning on the genes that can trigger the diseases of our generation.

When I first started drinking celery juice it was because it was recommended so highly for EBV. The information was that Epstein-Barr virus (EBV) is the cause of so-called autoimmune conditions like Hashimoto's. If you research in the medical journals, the researchers agree that infections like EBV can be the trigger for RA, lupus, Sjogren's syndrome and a list of other autoimmune disorders. Just go check out the research on PubMed while it is still available. I say that because sometimes valuable information is slowly depleted from our reach. They say that these autoimmune diseases are a dysregulation of EBV that causes synovial inflammation, which for RA is localized in the joints. Sounds a lot like other chronic pain related syndromes, right? EBV infects more than 95% of the world's population. Think about that for a minute.

Another study was done to show how pregnant women in Japan were exposed to a variety of chemicals and heavy metals that were then transferred to their fetus. Phthalates, perfluorinated compounds, and several heavy metals were what they found in the fetus, although there were high levels of phthalates, perfluorinated compounds, pesticides, polybrominated diphenyl ethers, and heavy metals in the maternal blood, cord blood, maternal urine and amniotic fluid in the women studied.

My parents gave me horrible oral bacteria as an infant, and at age five when I went to the dentist for the first time I had six cavities. My entire life I had many cavities, and then I had all of the mercury fillings replaced. However when looking at the difference between the plastic composite resins (bisphenol A also called BPA), or the metal amalgam fillings I had containing mercury it's hard to say where the most damage will come from. I have to believe that with the endotoxins I am better off without the heavy metals, although mice injected with BPA showed increased endotoxic activation. BPA may be a trigger for infectious autoimmune inflammatory reactions, as well. (16) That makes more sense that we need to figure out how to reduce sugar, and increase oral health good microbes.

We get so many toxins from our parents, and then through fillings, contact lens solution, eating some tuna, power plants, chlorine in the water, lead and the topper, vaccines. Then we give our children in the United States more vaccines over the first year of their life than I think any child should have to be exposed to. Especially powerful when we start to consider the genetic inability to detoxify many of those toxins including heavy metals. As well streptococci, gut dysbiosis, drugs like antibiotics, gastric acid and bile deficiency can all also play a part with heavy metal toxicity. I am not anti-vax, and my daughter has had all of her vaccines except for one. I just believe that the current schedule is overabundant and should be further looked at.

We aren't just being exposed to more chemicals since the last large war, but we're eating more commercially processed meats than we ever have before. The food we eat is modified, including our corn, soy, sunflower, rice and wheat. Farmers put on full toxic uniforms and spray down their crops with fungicides, insecticides and pesticides. We eat these crops, and more importantly for many of us is that our meat eats these crops. Then we box everything up in chemicals, and add in artificial colors, flavors and preservatives to keep us coming back for more. And now we have a plethora of plant based and lab created meat coming into the markets that are high in inflammatory ingredients. All of these cause more gut dysfunction, which causes more of those histamine 2 drugs. Looking at the data it is interesting that all of this has run directly parallel to the increase in MS, Crohn's, even Type 1 diabetes and other diseases.

All of these things are directly related to the mucosal lining in our gut, and with all of that leaky gut going on; those endotoxins can cross the gut mucosa into the bloodstream. Leaky gut is the red flag signal for autoimmune diseases. Our protection is one cell thick. If it is true that EBV can infect the gastric mucosa at the time of primary infection (17), then are we leaky from birth causing all of these other problems?

Heavy metal elements and their compounds seem to bind easily to sulfur and sulfur compounds, so what do you do if you don't deal with sulfur very well? First off, you have to have enough glutathione for the sulfur detoxification process.

But glutathione isn't just important for detoxification. Have you ever heard of glycation? This is a natural process in which the sugar in your bloodstream attaches to proteins. What it forms is harmful new molecules called advanced glycation end products. This is the process we see when we start seeing aging signs on our skin. This process shows up using special cameras as a fluorescent light. When the camera is used to take a photo of a child's skin, it's a very dark photo. Take a photo of someone of my age, and it is really lit up. Since glucose makes our skin cells abnormal; and then it creates free radicals, it is important to note that too much glycation can affect what type of collagen you can build and the amount of elastin your skin has. That is why those with diabetes often age prematurely. Polyphenols have powerful antioxidants that help protect cells from glycation. One more reason for a rich polyphenol diet.

Glutathione isn't just about correcting sulfur, it is sulfur. Glutathione contains sulfur compounds. That there is the catch-22 of this game of detoxification. The one most important detoxification pathway for those environmental toxins and carcinogens and most of the toxins excreted in the bile and the kidneys is what we call glutathione conjugation. Being able to eliminate those heavy metals is dependent upon having enough glutathione. We need some amino acids like methionine and cysteine as well to complete this conjugation. You get that methionine from eating nuts, meat, shellfish, dairy and legumes. Homocysteine is also an amino acid.

I have mentioned my CBS mutation in regards to my inadequate ability to deal with high levels of sulfur. CBS is an enzyme, Cystathionine-Beta-Synthase. Its job is to convert homocysteine into cystathionine, which is then converted into cysteine. This is our body's only mechanism for removing those sulfur containing amino acids when we have too much. If you have MTHFR you may have learned a little about homocysteine. MTHFR is that lack of the enzyme to convert all of the synthetic folic acid we are eating into the folate form that the body's metabolic pathways require. The MTHFR c677T homozygous mutation is the one that causes elevated levels of homocysteine. However if you have the a1298c mutation you may think you don't have to worry. What we have all been told is that a1298C mutations do not display elevated homocysteine unless they are combined with c677T. Yet research done in India in 2005 showed that homocysteine levels were significantly elevated in individuals adhering to a vegetarian diet or having MTHFR a1298C polymorphism. (20)

Homocysteine is the starting molecule of this metabolic pathway. However homocysteine also occupies a key location in the methionine cycle, and occupies one folate (carbon) cycle. This together is that methylation cycle. Methionine is one of the amino acids that are becoming a key to some very therapeutic cancer therapies, where medically blocking folate receptors has been used. Methionine is a sulfur-containing essential amino acid that is one of the nine provided to the body by food.

Soil that has been highly fertilized again and again, along with the impact of acid rain has been shown to create high levels of sulfur. For those of you that drink well water, or fancy San Pellegrino carbonated mineral water, you are drinking extra sulfur. It may be a wellness choice worth taking on, but knowing means you may want to start slow in the process. Cows, sheep and even horses have died from high levels of sulfur in their feed and water. For us, it is in that CBS pathway that these sulfur amino acids are removed. Yet just like with copper, those of us that are sulfur sensitive seem to crave them, because of the quick boost we get before the chaos ensues. Now you see the complexity of a balance in our diets. And now that sulfur can be in your plants from high fertilization, and it's in those cruciferous vegetables, mushrooms, dairy and meat, what are you supposed to eat in order to keep detoxing naturally, while not becoming sulfur toxic?

Research shows that frequent consumption of milk, yogurt, cold breakfast cereals, peppers, and cruciferous vegetables and intakes of dietary folate and riboflavin but not vitamins B12 and B6 are inversely associated with serum total homocysteine concentrations in the US population. (21) I feel that this is all wrapped into the methylation pathway, a nation overloaded with methylfolate-rich and folic-rich blood, and the growing expression of genetic mutations. The truth is we need the micronutrients. You can cycle these foods in and out of your diet while using items to help reduce the problems associated with this poorly functioning pathway. Using molybdenum, the right type of B12 and some yucca powder can all be helpful, as can reducing the amount of those foods you are eating. I also have found the use of glycine can help, but again, not too much because part of the detox pathway is the methionine and glycine removes methionine from the body. Depending on what you are eating, glycine can be synthesized by the body as well. So we really are what we eat. Since methionine contains that Sulphur atom, which can be involved in binding to atoms such as those heavy metals, nutrients matter.

Glutathione is supportive to lower inflammation, and yet NF-kB activates inflammation (as well as cells growth) and thus, disease. We need both of these functioning in our bodies to respond to toxins and disease. When NF-kB is activated you may see higher levels of depression, anxiety, leptin disruption, and more. So we need NF-kB, but we don't need too much. One of the simplest ways to inhibit NF-kB is to eat more fruits and veggies that contain those good phytochemicals and getting those micronutrients.

Plants cannot survive without glutathione, as well, and so don't let anyone tell you that plants aren't sources of glutathione. Apples, grapes, cucumber, peaches, lemons, mango, banana, butternut squash and zucchini all have both low levels of glutathione, and also low levels of sulfur. I also love artichoke hearts, which seems to fit the bill and I often rave about its higher protein levels you may be seeking.

One of the highest glutathione and sulfur containing plants is asparagus. Maybe that is why I have never really loved asparagus. New research conducted by several institutions, including the Cancer Research UK Cambridge Institute in the United Kingdom showed that Asparagine, an amino acid derived from a varied range of foods like asparagus, helps deadly breast cancer to spread. (22) I don't know if it was because of the increase in genetic mutations that deal with this pathway; however I do find it interesting.

As you have found, I love me some turmeric. I promised to talk more about my favorite spice. Ayurveda considers turmeric to be nature's most powerful healer. Turmeric also inhibits inflammatory NF-kB. Researchers have found that the curcumin found in turmeric can assist in restoring adequate levels of glutathione and improve the activity of glutathione enzymes. Another one of my favorite spices, ginger, due to its component gingerol, has also been shown to exert anti-inflammatory effects through mediation of NF-κB. I just recently read that traditional Chinese medicine uses curcumins to treat depression and stress. Curcumin is an extract created from turmeric. This is supported by the fact that curcumins reversed impaired hippocampal neurogenesis which is responsible for stress, depression and anxiety. Maybe my morning tea does create pure happiness.

During neurogenesis, which is a process of neural cell formation, NFκB signaling mediates the effect of numerous niche factors. Most of the research I have seen in this area goes way over my geek abilities; however, what I know is that there may be a link of NFκB signaling defects to various neurodevelopmental disorders. Currently the belief is that immune and inflammatory responses are to blame, but NFκB signaling mediates most actions of these immune and inflammatory factors.

Also, in regards to curcumin, it is an indirect activator of the Aryl Hydrocarbon Receptor (AhR) The AhR is a protein best known for its role in mediating toxicity. When AhR are activated by a pollutant, they trigger the expression of genes controlling reactions like oxidative stress and inflammation. AhR mediates the toxic effects of items like dioxins. Dioxins are a group of toxic chemical compounds. A 2010 study showed that dioxins changed Igs and C levels and suppressed humoral immunity in rats. (23) The harmful effects of this were prevented by curcumin when given at doses of 100 mg/kg/day. It is thought that this effect of curcumin may be due to AhR, but they say more studies are needed. Although in 2014 another study showed the protective effect of curcumin against heavy metals-induced liver damage. (24) I think for myself, turmeric daily is helpful in more ways than I can understand. Some of you may find that turmeric isn't as effective because it can raise thiol levels. Always remember that we are all built just a little bit different.

So now, it's no secret that I start my day with that glorious turmeric and ginger tea. It has been a part of my routine for several years, although I did get out of the habit right around the time I started having issues with ammonia. I morphed into drinking my green tea every morning. However, I have learned that I need to have the support of my organic turmeric and ginger as a must daily. Yes, green tea extract also suppresses NFκB activation and inflammatory responses; however it also blocks the absorption of some essential B vitamins. So I make sure I don't have it until my body has had the chance to use those booster micronutrients, and I don't actually have green tea every day. I cycle it. One serving of matcha green tea has 34 mg of free amino acids, including L-methionine.

8

Moldy

As you move into using more herbs the biggest thing you have to be aware of, and with any grains you decide to keep in your diet, is the mold.

I had never heard of Alternaria alternata until I started really delving into what could be at the root trigger of my latex reactions. When I hit that high in the summer season in July, the year of creating something new was triggered in a very bad way. Talk about manifesting. I created something very new. At first, remember, I thought it may be that keto rash I had read so much about and dealt with in the past. However, I really wasn't eating enough fats or low enough in carbohydrates to be that deep into ketosis. I really did learn my lesson before, and I was working in my higher carb, plant heavy version.

Alternaria alternata is a mold/fungus that has been recorded causing leaf spot and other diseases on over 380 various plants. I didn't know until I started down this research path that A. alternata is recognized as an important allergen with airborne spores and mycelial fragments (the vegetative part of a fungus or fungus-like bacterial colony) being responsible for the allergic symptoms in individuals with rhinitis or bronchial asthma. Asthma is also something that until the last several years has been a thorn in my side. I was on daily inhaled steroids when I was pregnant with my daughter because if mama doesn't get oxygen then neither does the baby.

A study was done where dust samples were collected from a bed, sofa, or a chair, and from the bedroom, living room, and kitchen floors as data as part of the National Survey of Lead and Allergens in Housing. What they found was that exposure to A alternata in US homes is associated with active asthma symptoms. This was in 2006. Later in 2014 they dug deeper and what they found was that only eight recombinant single allergens from three mold species are available for molecular allergy diagnosis of mold sensitization. This showed that the major allergen in Alternaria alternata-sensitized individuals was potential cross-reactivity to mold, food and natural latex allergens.

So when I think about this in terms to my body, I had to go down the rabbit hole again of research and I ended with food. I have listened to Dave Asprey talk about mycotoxins and just let it flow over me for years. Multipassionistas, it all feels disconnected until you realize it is all relevant to your process. Now I realized I needed to listen. Alternaria toxins can be found in grains when drying in the field and harvest are delayed by rain, high humidity, or early frost, mostly in sorghum. Right now as I am writing this soy farmers are holding their soybeans in silos hoping in six months or more the prices will increase. Post-harvest occurrence of Alternaria species in fruits and vegetables is more common because the moisture content remains high after harvest, and have been seen in apples all the way into the core, oranges, tomatoes, alfalfa, dry bog cranberries, carrots, eggplant, blueberries and bell peppers. It has also been found in nuts, including peanuts, hazelnuts, and pecans, papaya, wheat and cold-stored meat and spices. In my head as I am reading this I keep thinking nightshades, latex, and about autoimmune diet protocols and thinking things are syncing up. This also may explain why when I have these fruits and veggies after they have picked at their prime, flash frozen and then low temp dehydrated, I just have no problems with them. Infection requires germination.

This mold is also found one of the common molds isolated in grapes and responsible for the spoilage of wine because they produce anti-yeast metabolites. Being that this is a high mold in plant-based spoiled foods, it makes me think that it is probably in a lot of plant-based packaged foods and preservatives we don't even know about. Personally, I don't like oaked wines. I don't know if they are at higher risk of molds, but they just don't create the happiness I see in my friends when they are strolling through wineries here and in Napa.

Up to 80% of infections in the body affecting the body systems are associated with biofilm formation. We talked earlier a little bit about this, from infants and beyond. One thing I have found is that they are starting to use surfactant as a tool to reduce mold on foods, and in studies targeting biofilms in the body. Will this come back to bite us in the butt later on? I don't know. Like I said, as humans we are quite pretty but often very stupid. I do know that molds generally do not grow in or even on the surface of biofilms. Alternaria is not a common colonizer of biofilms, and so I don't see it as being a great impact overall in these current studies to remove these infections from our foods. However we won't know until we know. Research in anything related to the underground food movement is slow, at best.

Part of this latest latex reactivity cycle started in the perfect storm. I had my haircut and starting using hair spray again. I bought a bunch of fancy makeup and was getting all done up. I was using a facial oil that comes from a latex-based fruit, and I started using CBD oil for my joint pain (without stopping the incoming nightshade foods that I love).

Cannabis use is associated with sensitization to specific allergens, including mold, dust mites, plants, and cat dander. Alternaria alternata frequently blights marijuana and produces a toxin called alternariol, which is also high in sunflower. Sunflower is my most serious food allergy. Since up to 70% of mold allergy patients have skin test reactivity to Alternaria, the question is a chicken and the egg. So I have an alternariol allergy or an alternaria allergy as the core of my allergy bundle? What a question, right? And the worst part is that mold thrives in a heavy metal environment.

In both Germany and the US, research was done that showed that invading microbes like mold will set up house in the body compartments with the highest levels of toxic metals. It wasn't until I was writing this book that I connected the fact that I had spent a vast amount of my childhood sleeping next to a wall that was hiding toxic black mold. Then when I first lived in the Seattle area I was dealt with the worst sinus infections of my life. My allergist called Seattle the city of mold. I have found this is a national crisis. The steroids didn't do a thing to make me better, nor did the antibiotics they prescribed.

Having had six cavities the first time I went to the dentist when I was five probably means I still have a lot of mercury in my body that I am trying to detox, and in the surrounding tissues. Dietrich Klinghardt, MD, Ph.D said that, "The teeth jawbone, Peyer's patches in the gut wall, the ground system (connective tissue) and the autonomic ganglia are common sites of metal storage and the place where microbes thrive. Furthermore, those bodily areas are also vasoconstricted and hypoperfused by blood, nutrients, and oxygen, which foster the growth of anaerobic germs, molds, fungi, and viruses." So I lived in a house with black mold as a child, and then moved into a city with lots of mold, all while loving my nori and having a kajillion fillings in my mouth. So although years later I have gotten rid of the fillings, but not the mold and heavy metal leftovers.

The big things I have challenged in my body are really about trying to change the way it reacts, and reducing the hyperactive mast cell responses. We do know that mast cells activation is often triggered by mold. Mercury and aluminum are also big mast cells triggers. Do you use deodorant? See where I am going with this?

So what else can you put in your heavy metal arsenal? I was told that chlorophyll and celery juice neutralizes ammonia. Liquid chlorophyll is a wonderful support that is low in sulfur. Chlorophyll can help neutralize excess ammonia caused by eating those sulfur-rich foods. Eating enough of those leafy greens like baby spinach, rainbow chard or wrapping your foods into a big collard leaf is a great way to help your body reap the rewards of chlorophyll. A lot of people add cilantro into their diet to detox heavy metals, but when you react to sulfur, it isn't always the best choice. Cilantro can also increase thiols, which is one part sulfur. My experience is that a small amount of pressed cilantro is best, and has not caused me any problems.

No matter where you Google, you are going to find different answers. This book is also not a one size fits all, but rather an introduction to trying to figure out your own nutritional path. The things that we can all relate to are that too much inflammation is not great, and too many toxins are bad. Start from there, and move your happiness forward.

9

In the Soil

Someone once said to me that we aren't as smart as we are fast. I think about these types of sayings and laugh and shake my head in acknowledgment of the truth. We act, before we have answers, and we are just un-smart enough to sometimes choose the wrong solutions. I jumped into the vegan diet before I had any idea about the fats I was lacking. I jumped into the vegan diet before I knew what was in and what was lacking in our soil. I jumped into the vegan diet without the understanding that I had genetic mutations and needed some supplementation that I wasn't going to get from my daily diet. All of this has a lot to do with some of the changes I have made in my life, one of which is not to stop being vegan. You thought I was going in a different direction, right? Well I find that plant based is what sings to me, calls to me, and heals me.

As well as our soil being very high in sulfur, it's also high in toxins causing aluminum toxicity. Who loves avocados? (Every keto and paleo kid in the bunch raises their hands) I read a study that was conducted to document nutrient and pesticide concentrations in storm water runoff from nursery, citrus, and avocado production sites, and to assess the potential for groundwater contamination with nutrients from these sites by measuring nutrient concentrations in the soil water below the root zone of these crops. I have been teaching this in small groups, and hoping to see the information get out there. But the lobby to eat avocados is strong.

Leaching of nitrate and pesticides can contribute to groundwater contamination. The results in the study suggested that potential groundwater contamination with nutrients from citrus, avocado, and nursery sites may be as much of a concern as nutrient runoff for these operations.

So now we also have less rainfall and hotter summers, so you may think that the storm water runoff doesn't matter as much. But these samples were taken all the way down into the water table below the roots. And soils formed under low rainfall conditions tend to be basic with soil pH readings around 7.0. Intensive farming over a number of years with nitrogen fertilizers or manures can result in acidic soil. In the wheat-growing regions of Kansas and Oklahoma, for example, they have soil pH of 5.0 and below, and has resulted in aluminum toxicity in wheat.

Beyond that, most of the country, and from studies across all of the UK, we know our soil is lacking selenium. Selenium has the ability to reduce the toxicity of heavy metal ions like cadmium and mercury. Over and over again, selenium keeps coming into my messages as something I desperately needed. However just like we've talked about, not enough is just as bad as too much. Those with the CBS mutation often have a hard time eliminating selenium, and it may be dependent on the form of selenium used or even other dysfunctional pathways. This is where that functional doctor can be such a huge help in your healing journey.

There are three types of selenium supplements. First is the regular form of selenium that is in most multivitamins. The second is called Selenomethionine, also called either L-selenomethionine or selenium monomethionine. This form is considered a more bioavailable form of selenium. When looking at some of the therapeutic studies using selenium, you may also stumble upon selenium-enriched yeast. This yeast is grown on selenium and predominantly consists of selenomethionine. Research shows that selenium yeasts represent probably the best absorbed form of this element. It is generally produced by fermentation of baker's yeast grown in a selenium-rich medium. This is considered to be an organic food-form selenium supplement. What happens in this is that virtually all of the selenium structurally substitutes for sulfur in the amino acid methionine thus forming selenomethionine via the same pathways and enzymes that are used to form sulfur-containing methionine. Selenium yeast is capable of increasing the activity of the selenoenzymes. As well, its bioavailability has been found to be higher than that of inorganic Selenium sources in all but one study.

The concern as I said before is with our genetics, could we be at risk of selenium toxicity? What I have found is research that was done on intervention studies with Selenium yeast have shown the benefit of this form in cancer prevention, on the immune response and on HIV infection. (24) Of about one dozen supplementation studies, none has shown evidence of toxicity even up to an intake level of 800 µg Se/d over a period of years.

So I looked at the study of Finnish men, they seem to do all of the cool studies in Scandinavia. My Viking ancestors are something pretty amazing. They looked at the effects of selenium yeast, selenite, and selenate. Our tissues are particularly sensitive to changes in selenium supply including red blood cells, our kidney and muscles. And what they keep finding is that organic food-form selenium is more effective at increasing glutathione peroxidase activity compared with selenomethionine. That activity has everything to do with selenium, and without it we may contribute to increased free radicals over our lifetime.

So why haven't we been concerned about the lack of selenium in the soil? Perhaps it is because plants don't require it, just humans and animals. The UK, Australia, New Zealand, Denmark and the Atlantic Region of Canada are all dealing with selenium deficient soil. When we aren't getting selenium, that's a not so good idea. We become deficient. However if the farmers are adding a toxic selenium to the soil, and into their animals, we are at an even bigger risk of selenium toxicity. It is as important to know what isn't in the soil, as what is.

Selenosis, or selenium toxicity, can cause neurological problems, damage our nerves causing peripheral neuropathy. There are over 100 types of peripheral neuropathy, and the diseases that I often think about in regards to idiopathic peripheral neuropathy include MS, CFS and CF. You can get genetic testing for hereditary neuropathies, but not for those that just come along for the ride. There is however a high association of MTHFR gene c677T mutation with diabetic peripheral neuropathy and diabetic retinopathy. (25) Most studies focus on hyperhomocysteinemia as associated with diabetic neuropathy, and this new information on the MTHFR mutation being associated is fantastic for all of the people wondering where this came from. Knowing that you may have a predisposition is often just what you need to know in order to take preventive measures.

On top of selenium, Dr. Weil has recommended taking glucose-tolerance factor (GTF) chromium. Chromium is involved in the action of insulin, and so highly advertised for those with metabolic syndrome. GTF chromium is chromium that has been chemically bound to natural Vitamin B3 (nicotinic acid or niacin). This form functions as a glucose tolerance factor, and is very different than chromium picolinate.

High amounts of chromium can be toxic to humans and to plants. Lead, cadmium, and chromium are found in many of the chemical fertilizers used today. A toxicity report on formulants and heavy metals in glyphosate-based herbicides and other pesticides. They looked at glyphosate alone and 14 of its formulations. They identified arsenic, chromium, cobalt, lead and nickel in the pesticide formulations. (26) If you consider that all of the major pesticides used around the world are glyphosate-based herbicides, that's pretty scary. Ingestion of chromium can cause kidney and liver damage, stomach ulcers, vomiting, hemolysis, heart problems and possibly reproductive problems. (27) So even if you are growing organic vegetables, what soil you are growing in matters. At my home we grow in raised gardens so we can control the soil, and in urban indoor gardens so that there is no soil to worry about.

As a trace mineral, do you need to supplement with chromium or not? Chromium picolinate interferes with the absorption of thyroid medications. I can't find any information on GTF chromium, but I wouldn't recommend taking it with your thyroid medication either. In fact, the only thing I can really find is that GTF chromium is said to help improve the conversion of T4 to T3. We honestly don't even know enough to say what a healthy recommendation of chromium supplementation should be. The University of Maryland Medical Center says that up to 90 percent of Americans may not be getting enough chromium through food. If there is so much going into the soil, why aren't we able to use it? What is it bound to?

So what does the thyroid have to do with happiness? Thyroid hormones have a direct connection to mental health, including issues like anxiety and depression. One meta-analysis suggests that T3 may accelerate antidepressant response in patients with treatment-resistant depression. Likewise, T3 augmentation can improve depressive symptoms in patients without subclinical hypothyroidism whose depression did not fully respond to selective serotonin reuptake inhibitors (SSRIs). (28)

One item I found is that my thyroid levels always came back not too far off and so I didn't jump into the idea that I needed to support my thyroid. This was a mystery because I had so many symptoms that were associated with a struggling thyroid. When you are in ketosis you may see a slightly lower T3 level, but you need to test your Reverse T3. A study, published in Diabetes, Obesity and Metabolism, found that a ketogenic diet resulted in lowered T3 levels and raised Reverse T3 levels in healthy subjects. Without enough active T3, you can see a whole herd of problems. Your T3 is your body's energy generator. Ferritin is your body's gasoline. Imagine what is happening to those with both not enough functional T3 and not enough gasoline. It isn't that you have parenthooditis, you are truly lacking energy.

You can also see this higher Reverse T3 level when you are doing Intermittent Fasting (IF) or putting your body into starvation mode by not eating enough calories. So there is this cycle that starts to happen where you cannot eat too many calories because you are not moving enough, and yet you are creating the perfect storm for your thyroid. So while you may not have responded in the past to a mixed T4/T3 prescription, it may be that you just need more T3 to help your body reset. Energy is ATP (the body's primary energy source) and decreased ATP availability during your heavy dieting or fasting could impair this T4 uptake by the liver. Remember that your liver is the main organ responsible for this conversion of T4 to T3, and so make sure you take the time to support your liver function if you want to have a better functioning body. Beyond this, remember that your body doesn't like to not get those macronutrients and micronutrients. Working with someone like myself to help you get highly dense nutritional values during the day while slowly increasing your energy is going to be vital.

One more note on ATP for those that are active. I always tell my athletes, especially weight lifters, to have their ferritin levels tested. Without your iron levels in a good range you cannot effectively produce ATP. If you want to see a measureable decrease in your performance and capacity, and reduced VO2max, then skip checking your ferritin levels.

On the opposite side is those that store iron due to genetic mutations. When you have a genetic disorder where you store iron in your organs, you can see an increased risk of diabetes, arthritis, liver inflammation, thyroid function and even sexual dysfunction. It can really complicated treating your thyroid disease, so get your genetics tested and then if you have the hemochromatosis gene, talk to your functional support team about how to work on treatment. It is important to note that substantial deposition of iron in the thyroid gland is a frequent autopsy finding in patients with genetic haemochromatosis. We're even seeing iron accumulating in the brain as we age, and that has been linked to motor and cognitive dysfunction in the elderly. Green tea catechins have been researched as brain-permeable, and can be used as a non-toxic iron chelators to "iron out iron" from the brain. The off side of this is that you should take it separated from not just your thyroid medication, but away from your folate, and iron supplementation as it will also attach to these and pull that out of the body. If you are trying to conceive this is very essential to get those healthy folate foods and whole food supplements.

All of these types of diets when not done properly can then suppress your hypothalamic-pituitary-thyroid axis. This system regulates your metabolism and will support how your body deals with stress. It is the response of low thyroid hormones that tells your pituitary to stimulate the thyroid gland to produce more. A recent (March 2008) peer reviewed study published in the Journal of American Neurotoxicology and Teratology states that only small to moderate amounts of pesticides in rats cause excessive weight gain by damaging brain structures like the hypothalamus and the pituitary (Lassiter, 2008). You truly are what you eat. Eat that sexy beast!

Your body makes an extremely important hormone called MSH (Melanocyte Stimulating Hormone). MSH is produced in the hypothalamus by Leptin, and it controls nerve, hormone, cytokine functions, skin and mucus membrane defenses, and the production of endorphins and melatonin. If your brain cannot hear Leptin, and is therefore "Leptin Resistant," you will eventually become MSH deficient (Shoemaker, 2005). Leptin tells your brain what to do. So what happens if your fearful lizard brain runs its own show? That is correct; your lizard brain (brain stem) is where the leptin hormone becomes blocked from reaching the leptin receptors. This means that you will keep eating without feeling satisfied.

If you do not recognize how important essential micronutrients, healthy fats, breathing, mindfulness, joy, grace are in the grand scheme of your body finding its way back to the healthy space, you will have missed the greatest item in this entire book. If you continue to live in the same way, without asking your body what is going on, what it needs, what makes it happy... this is your end.

10

Being Ketogenic

A few years ago the University of Saskatchewan came out with research showing that methylglyoxal is a cause of type 2 diabetes. Because of this you are seeing a wave of joy across the keto and fasting communities. There is a lot of information out there on methylglyoxal, none of which your average person can understand. The important part to understand is that methylglyoxal is toxic to our cells. Diabetics have an increased concentration of both sugars, and methylglyoxal in their blood. Ketone acetoacetate, the metabolite that is released from fat-metabolism and is one of the ketone bodies, can capture and inhibit methylglyoxal. When you pee on a ketone urine strip, you are testing for acetoacetate that has been made in the liver from fatty acids. It is used for energy when glucose isn't available. It is the beta-hydroxybutyrate (BHB) that is the prevalent ketone in ketoacidosis, and can rise in diabetic ketoacidosis. Acetone, the third and least abundant ketone, and is spontaneously formed from the breakdown of acetoacetate. It is also the ketone body that most say triggers the keto rash.

Acetoacetate is the first ketone the body produces, which is converted into BHB and acetone. If you do short stints of a ketogenic diet or true fast, you will have mostly acetoacetate in your bloodstream. After three weeks of either of those you will have mostly BHB in your bloodstream. This is why I like the idea of either daily intermittent fasting, or small bursts of my plant heavy ketogenic diet with weeks of refeeding in order to reset the ketone production. I will fast for sixteen hour a day on the average day, usually starting by 6 PM. This allows my body to have the entire night to go through the natural functions of repair and renewal. It also allows me the benefits of keto without the harsh dietary extremes of the average keto plan.

So this is where I came up with the idea for the fourteen day Ketolicious Reset that I could alternate with the ten day shredding program I had been running with the customers. I find in this day and age, a good focus on cleansing the liver and the gallbladder is essential more often than once a year. My January groups are filled to the brim, but just focusing on detoxification during January isn't going to cut it. The liver and gallbladder are vital for your digestion and immune system.

Your liver is responsible for filtering and neutralizing harmful substances and unmetabolized items from your body. It has 500 metabolic jobs, which it cannot perform optimally when overburdened with toxins.

To have a healthy liver and be free of those sugar cravings, you need healthy bile flow, and this can only happen with a healthy gallbladder. Your gallbladder breaks down the fats you eat, which is why I recommend using bitters when you first introduce changes and increase plant based fats in your diet. If you get indigestion when you eat, this is the perfect program for you because you are eating foods that seasonally cleanse the gallbladder. Not only do the liver and gallbladder have a physical job but your organs are also usually attached to an emotion block.

LIVER = ANGER
GALLBLADDER = RESENTMENT

Allow yourself to let go of daily emotional baggage, and use whatever physical and emotional tools you can in this program to release the toxic burden, emotionally and spiritually, and find some freedom. When was the last time you said this: I'm going paleo. I'm going vegan. I'm going to start P90X ... again? I'm going to be more active with the kids. I'm going to stop eating ALL the chocolate and drinking ALL the wine (diet soda... you get the idea). I am going to stop looking at EVERYONE else and start being thankful for all that I am. I have worked with a lot of people on their subtle energy bodies. The problem is that we get our chakras balanced and our aura in tune, and then you pick up the cell phone and hit that little social media icon. You look at the life you wish you had, grab that big old glass of wine, a second cupcake, and put on the stretchy pants. That's our truth!

You want this, but we don't connect to it! We want it, but we don't know what's going on internally that's blocking all of this! I'm giving you hints, but you are the one that has to stop and listen to your body. You are the only one that knows what's deeply seeded internally that's blocking your body from finding some real happiness.

When you don't think you know, focus on what you do know. How do you feel when you eat that avocado? How do you feel when you start getting into ketosis? How does this supplement make you feel? How does this food impact your energy? How does this exercise impact your waistline? Even the scary question, how does this person make me feel? We know that our body is like a machine. It needs nutrients, oxygen and sleep to work functionally. If you have kids, or dogs, or a snoring spouse I may not be able to do a lot for the longevity of your sleep. However we know that in life if we want anything we have to consciously choose it, and that is true for everything. This idealism, the right combination of macrostax and micronutrients can help you choose better when you need to most in order to feel like you desire. I want you to be able to choose how you want to feel, and what you want to be regardless of what's happening around you. As I have shared, our machine runs on mostly plant based nutrients, energetic vibrations and the highest power, love. Eat well, be mindful, and choose love.

Science gave me the answer when I needed it most. Really it did. I was reaching for information on alcoholism because I have a long line of alcoholism in my ancestry and super woven into my genetics. What I found was that lack of the good hormones in the brain is the answer to bad choices. But with those leaky guts, and negative microbiome, and the pain and agony of the (place your own horrible allergy creating food here) we just can't do it. Autoimmune, genetic mutations, food allergies, and so much more are woven into mine, and your body, but awareness and simplicity of nutrition offers us all the answers. Isn't it funny that we live in a world full of food choices, but most of them have no nutritional value to offer our bodies?

What if you could do something so simple that you'd lean into that happier mindset, and thus strengthen your certainty and faith when moving into those other choices? Sometimes it takes something as simple as what we can offer you, and that makes so many other differences in our life, and your gut. It is really hard to go after your actual desires if you are curled up on the couch feeling like garbage. While food and micronutrients may not manifest your destiny, it will give you the space and awareness to be open to the choices.

Can food be your therapist, and not in a bad way? What about food as your comfort, and not in an "omg caller ID" sort of way. I am talking about getting as many plant-based micronutrients into your diet every single day to feed your body so that you can take care of the big stuff. Dr. Oz says we should automate our nutrition as much as possible, and I agree. But most of us get the same eight fruits & veggies over and over again, sometimes less when you switch over to a paleo, low carb or ketogenic diet. That has to stop.

You have to put plants first, and if you desire add in non-plants in a minimal amount. I understand that some people don't digest their vegetables very easily. Chewable digestive enzymes may help you, although I haven't quite figured that out because there are the people that seem to have no problem digesting animal proteins but just cannot eat kale. I guess they are cheering that kale is now the most highly pesticide-toxic vegetable in the nation. Still, I know that you need the plants, so find a way that you can have them that works with your gut. Maybe it's a green smoothie to make it almost predigested. Maybe you need to steam your veggies before you eat them. Maybe you need to consider what other enzymes your body needs support with. Maybe it is going to have to be the supplementation route.

My husband was once a baker. Can you imagine my gut in pain as I reached for another delightfully squishy rosemary sourdough slice? Xylanase is an enzyme used by bakers to soften or condition the dough. When I look at most of the digestive enzymes on the market they are created from plants in order to digest meats, fats, dairy, and legumes. However, what about this enzyme will help you eat the plants?

Interestingly enough, as humans we don't produce this enzyme. It's like we are fully mutant together. Finally there is something that everyone in the nation has in common. Don't worry, we'll find something else to argue about tomorrow. This enzyme breaks down the plant cell walls, and if we have the right gut bacteria, they will produce a little of it all on their own. It is naturally occurring for bacteria, or fungi, and even some insects. Carnivores would say this is a sign to eat bacon. I disagree, and say this is a sign that we don't eat enough plants to produce this so we must supplement it. This will help you to digest those high fibers, super food legumes. Any of those fibrous plant foods that you meat eaters struggle with, this secret enzyme is the key to help you and you need to consider it because remember that fiber is going to feed your good gut microbiota. I think it should be taken with a complex digestive enzyme, in order to get the most benefit for the buck.

As well as breaking down the food you have never liked to eat because of the way it made you feel, this enzyme can help degrade the biofilms that are dangerous to your body. I saw a study done back in 1997 in Denmark using enzymatic removal and disinfection of bacterial biofilms. The biofilms they used were Staphylococcus aureus, Staphylococcus epidermidis, Pseudomonas fluorescens, and Pseudomonas aeruginosa. Combining oxidoreductases with pectinase, arabanase, cellulase, hemicellulase, b-glucanase, and xylanase enzymes resulted in bactericidal activity as well as removal of the biofilm. This is why a complex digestive blend is what I like to recommend.

Cholesterol is one of the two fats that make up the cell membrane. These are the five main types:

Chylomicrons are very large particles that mainly carry triglycerides (fatty acids from your food). They are made in the digestive system and so are influenced by what you eat.

Very-low-density lipoprotein (VLDL) particles also carry triglycerides to tissues. But they are made by the liver. As the body's cells extract fatty acids from VLDLs, the particles turn into intermediate density lipoproteins, and, with further extraction, into LDL particles.

Intermediate-density lipoprotein (IDL) particles form as VLDLs give up their fatty acids. Some are removed rapidly by the liver, and some are changed into low-density lipoproteins.

Low-density lipoprotein (LDL) particles are even richer in pure cholesterol, since most of the triglycerides they carried are gone. LDL is known as "bad" cholesterol because it delivers cholesterol to tissues and is strongly associated with the buildup of artery-clogging plaque.

High-density lipoprotein (HDL) particles are called "good" cholesterol because they remove cholesterol from circulation and from artery walls and return it to the liver for excretion.

Those plant-based foods, such as coconut, palm oil and cocoa butter, do contain saturated fat.

A variety of plants also contain monounsaturated fat, which is good for your health. Monounsaturated fats can help reduce bad cholesterol and thus lower your risk of heart disease and stroke. Almonds, Brazil nuts and walnuts, for instance, have this kind of fat. Another food to try is tahini, a product made from sesame seeds. However, more and more people are finding that they are reactive to sesame. Keep that in mind and ease into it. Don't overlook the occasional avocado, organic extra virgin olive oil and low processed organic soybeans, all of which have the kind of beneficial fat you want to incorporate into your nutrition plan.

While some foods stand out as monounsaturated rock stars, others make their mark for having a high amount of polyunsaturated fat. This nutrient comes in two varieties: omega-3 and omega-6 fatty acids.

Food containing abundant amounts of these nutrients includes flaxseed, chia seeds and green leafy vegetables, such as broccoli. Walnuts pull double duty because they're rich in both mono- and polyunsaturated fats. The polyunsaturated fats can also lower your bad cholesterol and bring down your likelihood of developing heart disease, but they also provide essential nutrients that build and maintain your body's cells, including omega fatty acids. One reason it's so critical to eat foods containing these fatty acids is because the human body can't produce them on its own.

Your body relies on the liver to turn fat into cholesterol, which travels around the body through your blood.

Cholesterol comes in two forms. One protects the body, and the other has the potential to damage it. Problems arise when there's too much harmful cholesterol in your bloodstream, putting you at higher risk for cardiovascular disease. So, this is the heart of the matter: The dangerous cholesterol comes from saturated fat, and the good cholesterol comes from mono- and polyunsaturated fats. So don't let someone try to convince you that if you don't eat animals fats you won't be able to repair your cell membranes.

Eat plants with fat-soluble vitamins and healthy fat. One easy way to do this is to use healthy oils to prepare carrots, winter squash and mushrooms. You can also grab a handful of almonds or other nuts that are rich in unsaturated fats after your workout. You might find your muscles are a little less sore thanks to the fat's ability to reduce inflammation.

Choose freshly ground flaxseeds over flaxseed oil unless it is a part of the protocol you are working with. Both offer healthy fat, but the seeds come with the added benefit of fiber. Tip; mash the seeds, so you get the oil as well as the fibrous exterior. Lower high cholesterol by increasing polyunsaturated fat in your diet. This compound lowers all cholesterol, though both damaging and protective. Targeting harmful cholesterol levels with larger quantities of monounsaturated fats such as olive oil, or my favorite is algae oil is the best option. I use my algae oil every day in my morning Bulletproof tea.

When I was starting to have symptoms of sticky blood, I had my doctor run the tests. This was at least a year before Bob Harper had his heart attack. I was right on the money, and as a vegan my cholesterol was really high. Three months into my daily tea with oil, and a little citrus bergamot, and I reduced my bad cholesterol by 47 points and returned to a normal level. I rarely recommend fish oil these days because I am in love with the vegan omegas that I take every day. However, for those with genetically higher lipoprotein(a), those sticky blood platelets, you may not be getting enough EPA with your vegan supplementation. While we do know that for most people you are getting plenty with your diet plus the fact that your body metabolizes the 18-carbon ALA from plant foods to EPA and DHA. Studies have found that getting 1,800 mg/day of EPA over 6 months to 18 months reduces the level of the lipoprotein(a) and lipids in patients with vascular disease. (29) Current high does vegan supplements are using oils like sunflower oil, and I am not a fan of that for long term use of those types of oils. So you may either have to take lots of healthy plant based omegas throughout the day, or lean into a healthier (and pure) EPA that you can use for a time period to see how your body responds.

Getting into ketosis honestly is the easy part. If you start with about 50 - 75 net carbs daily, you will hit ketosis. If you are fatigued, make sure you are eating a little protein at each meal. The initial stimulating of your lymphatic system and supporting your liver, gallbladder and digestive system is the hard part. You have to do that so that once you start to remove toxins, which can be everything from those heavy metals to the molds, as you release from your fat cells is key. If you have worked alongside your liver and lymphatic system nicely you can move on to the introduction of some fats. Our cells require some fats for many reasons, but of course to repair. The idea of a plant-heavy ketogenic diet was not to get you into ketosis, but to get you into cellular change. In my "Beginners Guide to Keto" I cover not only what keto is, what the pitfalls are, but what you look for in terms of a need to return to the first steps of rejuvenation and resetting your body.

11

Return of the Woo Woo

To kick-start your body's natural metabolism and find your happy, you do have to start by eating the right portions of those macronutrients, getting enough calories and movement in order to eat. After that your body naturally cleanses and heals itself and those micronutrients from both supplementation and fruits and vegetables to help your system function smoothly.

Emotions can fuel your being in amazing ways, but for many of us its emotional eating that we turn to instead of learning to delve emotion. Rather than not eating because you are energetically awakening, we self-medicate with food in a low vibrational manner. I am one that had to deal with this learning curve, and so the student has become your teacher. I want you to know this truth because I want you to know there is no judgement and that I've been where you have.

We find ourselves eating when we feel angry, frustrated, and sad... and the whole realm of emotional urges. You may eat because of empathic urges, or just because you picked up the phone and heard someone that makes you feel anxious. Anxiety is a signal to your body, but we misread the message. It's like when I'm intuitively coaching someone, I have learned that the anxiety is actually a sign that there is some information that I really need to listen to. What do you need to listen to that you aren't? There is a reason why box breathing helps balance the nervous systems that impact anxiety. Your body is telling you to slow down and listen up. I want you to start tracking when you feel that feeling, daily. Tracking is a way to see something that we are struggling with in a different light. Those emotions are a key to something that you need to learn about, instead of eating them.

As a society we have become very dependent on sweet, sugary and refined foods for emotional satisfaction instead of healthier alternatives like nuts, seeds, fruits, and vegetables. In fact, 80% of children and 70% of adults are consuming fewer than five servings of vegetables and fruits per day, which could have a devastating effect on our collective mental well-being. A 2012 study of 80,000 people found that happiness and strong mental health is higher for those who consume daily portions of fruit and vegetables. We started this book with happiness, and happiness is the key to finding the light in your life.

Let me explain why. Serotonin is the neurotransmitter in the brain that produces a sense of calm and ease. Those that find ourselves with reduced serotonin levels, such as those with known bipolar disorder; the intake of carbohydrates produces tryptophan, which converts to serotonin and temporarily fills that void. So it makes some sense that people turn to food when they are feeling altered by emotions. Your brain runs on glucose or fats, and so most of us rely on carbohydrates to supply the energy it needs. The problem with binging on sugary foods is that it can mess with the brain's chemistry by alternating highs and lows. And when you feel those lows, then you're more likely to eat more. It's a vicious circle that we go through, this race with our emotions.

In a way, emotions are like an amazingly fierce racehorse. Your emotions are powerful and longing to be set free. As an emotional vibrational being your feelings are always in motion. We are energy, and energy doesn't stop. Our emotions crave this motion, and we try to rein them in, instead of going for a ride. When you lock your emotions in the stall, your racehorse will start kicking. And when you get too close to a kicking horse, you may get kicked!! Do you feel the energy you are passing along to those around you?

How many times have you kicked out when you felt like that? If you keep your emotions locked up, life will get pretty miserable at time. You'll end up battered and bruised, and so will those around you. And they'll end up believing that racehorses are bad. That is that tip of the cycle. Being bad opens us up to fear, shame, guilt, being unlovable and being then open to destroy our very own hearts.

Can you create a responsibility to own your emotions to let them be without judgement? Can you love without expectations? Can you eat without creating wrongness in it? This requires care and nurturing and time and effort and a commitment on your part. It means you have to stop the fight with your emotions, stop locking them up. I don't know what kind of relationship you have with your emotions, but I can make an educated guess. It's an adversarial one.

Emotions are bad and wrong and I'm weak and stupid for listening to them.

Emotions are the enemy.

I must learn to control my emotions.

Sound familiar? As you learn that emotions are not to be controlled, but are meant to be a guiding light to joy, easing you into a path of truth, and to everything you desire ... then your emotions will slowly move into a place of love. What amazing things will you create when you truly love yourself? It's like Wayne Dyer has said about an orange. If you squeeze an orange, you always get orange juice. No matter what type of pressure, time of day you will always get orange juice. When you don't like yourself, when you are angry, or sad, you will only see and give off those emotions blocking out the loving, joyful emotions. So I want you to work on noticing how your feelings attract like feelings.

Wholism is defined as an idea that different parts are all interconnected and cannot be understood without understanding the entire whole. We often forget the wholism when looking for our purpose and sharing our passion. We each have an amazing gift that we've been given, and it is the spark to the flame that will connect all of this vitality in your life.

While there are roughly 500 words in the English language to describe emotions, these all fall under one of these six categories: love, joy, anger, sadness, fear, and shame.

When thinking about how you feel you may describe joy using the words delight, blissful, ecstatic, and thrilled. When it's difficult to find the emotion, look up a list of light emotions and find the closest one.

So here's what to do now to start your journey:

1. Take a picture of yourself: I prefer doing this in something that reveals your middle. You can take the picture of yourself in the mirror, or you can have someone take it for you. You don't need to show anyone this picture. This is just for your own personal reference. If you follow the plan long term you will begin to see changes in your body, your skin will glow and you will feel more alive. And when you take your picture afterwards, you'll be pleasantly surprised with your before and after.

2. Weigh yourself: Get on your scale and take note of what you weigh right now. Write it down somewhere you will remember. If you want to write it down right here, here's a place to do so:

My Goodbye Weight: _____

Date: _____

You aren't losing weight, you are releasing toxins. That is why we do a photo and a weight. One of these two (most likely the photo) will show you what you have released in this journey. Also, weight is just a number on the scale, and nothing more. If you lose weight, you can find it later. So let's release those toxins and stored trauma energies that are no longer serving you well.

3. Write 3-4 sentences about how you feel right now. This is a great way to gain perspective. This doesn't need to be an impossible homework assignment. It just has to be a quick scan of how you feel emotionally and physically. Does anything hurt? When you get up in the morning? Do you have energy? Is it hard to sleep? Is it too easy to sleep!?! Be honest. You're on the track to fix these things that limit your health -- so it's great to have in mind exactly what you want to work on. Go ahead and write these sentences in a journal or in a word processing document. If you want, you can write it all here:

_____

_____

_____

_____

_____

_____

_____

_____

_____

_____

4. Set your targets: This is just the basics. Nothing set in stone. Writing clear concise targets of what you desire

(emotions, changes) allows you to focus on what you want. These thoughts will help you stay on track.

My targets for this change:

_____

_____

_____

I will know that I am aligned during and after this challenge because:

_____

_____

_____

What feelings could get in the way of my success, and what feelings do I desire:

_____

_____

_____

_____

_____

_____

How I can remove the emotional and physical roadblocks that could get in the way:

_____

_____

The actions I am committed to taking toward my success are:

If you haven't done so recently, you can go to your health practitioner and order a complete blood profile (CBC). This will measure many of your body's indicators of good or poor health - cholesterol, iron, calcium, etc. Also look at additional Lp(a) cholesterol (sticky blood) panels if you find you have moderately or high cholesterol for no reason. Most of this should be covered by most insurance plans (check with your provider) so it shouldn't cost you more than the co-pay. This is always great to do before you jump into anything new that relates to fitness and nutrition. You may even find that missing bit of the puzzle that has been underlying and causing all of this disconnection in our body. If you can, get those extra hormones, thyroid, ferritin, Vitamin D, homocysteine and omega levels.

If you don't know where you are, you won't make a good road map to get to where you want to be. You wouldn't leave Seattle to drive to Iowa without having an idea on how to get there. However you would know that you needed a car, and that the car needed fuel. You know that you have a body and it needs nutrition. You know that you have an energy that connects to how you feel, and so you have to nourish yourself to impact those emotions in many ways .I know that we often don't want to know where we are in our well journey, but it is something that matters so much. It's really why you are here!! You want more!

You want to release some of those feelings of hurt, anger, guilt, despair. Often how we release these emotions is by listening to our bodies, and recognizing that we are a part of something so much bigger. When we change our desires it vibrantly enhances our emotions. Did you hear that? How many times have you seen amazing changes in your life just because you were going with the flow of your desires? So I want you to think about the big picture. This is not about the scale, it's not about food. It's about love, happiness and reaching out to what you really want instead of stuffing down your feelings. If you don't allow your true emotional being to flow, you are blocking some amazing opportunities in your life. Let's change that.

As part of the change you are making I ask you to consider including a delicious whole food vegan shake daily. You may use this in the beginning of the day, as a snack or add to it and make it a meal. I find this important because it actually helps with your emotions because it helps balance your hormones and insulin response. It offers whole foods that are so very important to healing our bodies. These are foods you may have been lacking. So it's important that you use this tool every day as a part of your program.

At a recent panel discussion at the 2013 Institute of Food Technologists (IFT) Annual Meeting & Food Expo, Bonnie Kaplan of the University of Calgary said that getting supplementation can potentially be an alternative to increasing psychiatric medicines for symptom relief of anxiety and depression. My only guess is that it's all gut related. Our gut seems to be the center of the universe. In a series of studies, she found that people already diagnosed with having a mental disorder showed better mental functioning and well-being with a higher intake of these nutrients. She said that supplements can provide the mental energy necessary to manage stress, enhance mood, and reduce fatigue. I am giving you many extra plants in your day to help you with some of this emotional issue that is really nutritional deficiency so that you can work on the real emotional obstacles.

Systemically most detox programs are aggressive. Your body ends up moving toxins from one storage center to another because there is only so much your primary chimneys can do. When they can't release any more toxins they come through your skin. Ever hear someone say to you that they are feeling the detox because they have really broken out? That acne generally means they are really toxic. That means they need to increase the liver support, and maybe slow down the toxic release. These kinds or surges in our toxic levels are not healthy. You need something systemically healthy.

I love using additional support of flushing niacin a few hours before you workout or sauna, and then when you do workout and sauna taking some activated charcoal to bind to some of those toxins and help release them from the body for good. Again, don't take binders at the same time as you are taking medication or much needed supplementation. They will be bound. I have written about my sauna blanket on the Paleo Vegeo blog. It was created with low EMF and gives me everything I desired, as well as being easy to transport. If you don't have the space or cash for a large infrared sauna, this infrared sauna blanket is just what you have asked for.

This journey works because of the focus on wellness, and using the support of holistic products. I incorporate non-gmo, whole foods products because they are created in a manner that is tested, and tested again and continually clinically studied. Our lifestyle impacts more than 50% of our wellness, and its part of a new study area called Nutrigenomics.

Recent studies used microarray analysis while using non-gmo encapsulated whole foods to detect differences in gene expression before and after the intervention. In the subgroup of participants with high baseline CRP (inflammation), microarray analysis revealed that 1632 genes were differentially expressed after supplementation with the encapsulated concentrate. One thousand one hundred forty six genes were upregulated, while 486 genes were downregulated. From the genes that were significantly differentially expressed, several genes were identified that are involved in biologically-relevant signaling pathways, including: lipogenesis, NF-kB and AMPK pathways. These results showed that while all obese individuals are likely to gain some benefit from supplementation with these whole food products, those with high baseline systemic inflammation or blood lipids appear likely to obtain the greatest improvements. That's what made me stand up to attention with my lipoprotein(a) autoimmune issues that are tied to both inflammation and blood lipids, and with my lifetime of food and environmental allergies.

We are using whole foods, which of course the body is aligned to accept. You won't get healthy from taking a chemical. You are not synthetic. Nutrition that comes from whole foods comes from the life force of the plant, to fortify your system to reset your health. It comes from the soil, and it comes from the seed as well as the care.

A plant's secondary metabolites produce products that aid in the growth and development of plants but are not required for the plant to survive. Secondary metabolites facilitate the primary metabolites in plants. This primary metabolite consists of chemical reactions that allow the plant to live. In order for the plants to stay healthy, secondary metabolites play a pinnacle role in keeping all of the plants' systems working properly. A common role of secondary metabolites in plants is defense mechanisms. They are used to fight off herbivores, pests, and pathogens. Do you think you maybe are someone that is fighting off pathogens, chemicals, toxins, pollution? How about on a daily basis?

We need a daily detox and I know this not just from personal experience but by the education I have gained through my friends and mentors. It's difficult for your body to be in detoxification mode twenty hours a day. This process will ease you into healthier choices so that you aren't always fighting that muffin top and inflammation, and will give you the extra support to let your body detoxify in a manner that it was meant to, and at a pace that is healthy.

Don't think of this in terms of vitamins, but what we get from the whole food source. How would that impact your body and its ability to fight off pathogens, chemicals, toxins and more?

You need to get nutrition that comes from sustainable farming. Careful testing and independent experts ensure the natural purity of the finished products and foods. Not just looking for Non-GMO certifications, but organic and state-of-the-art facilities that meet or exceed highest food industry standards for blending, encapsulating, and packaging. For Pro Athletes standards that are reviewed and the NSA facilities inspected by NSF the public health and safety company matter, but the not-for-profit NSF certification is going to be essential for you with any additional supplementation.

Petrochemicals are chemicals made from crude oil and natural gas. There are over 4,000 products classified as petrochemicals. Petrochemicals and their byproducts, such as dioxin, are known to cause an array of serious health problems, including cancer and endocrine disruption (interference with hormones within your body). Endocrine disruptors interfere with growth, development, intelligence, and reproduction. The damage can be irreversible and be passed onto future generations.

Did you know that petrochemicals are found in most of your food products, personal care products, and household cleaning products?

Petrochemicals in conventional (non-organic) food often come from the fertilizer the food was grown in, the pesticides that were applied to it, the preservatives and artificial colors that were added to make it appealing, and the plastic the food was packaged and/or stored in. Petrochemicals are even used as a wax coating on such produce items as cucumbers, bell peppers, eggplant, potatoes, and citrus fruits.

Chemicals from the petroleum manufacturing process also enter our bodies through meat and dairy products. Chemicals such as pesticides and antibiotics tend to accumulate in milk and in animal flesh. In addition the manufacture and incineration of PVC (polyvinylchloride, #3) creates and disperses dioxins into the air and water. From there, they enter the food chain and accumulate in the fatty tissues of animals.

These chemicals are entering our bodies by being absorbed through the skin and scalp and then into our organs and tissues. Over time, these chemicals will affect your liver, brain, nerves, cause birth defects, infertility, severe allergies, acute asthma, and cancer.

There are over 80,000 chemicals used today and we don't even know the full effects they have on the human body.

You will never get rid of ALL of these chemicals, but when you focus on these sorts of changes, eliminations, and supplementation that can affect every cell of the body within 20 minutes and blood work can confirm the healing properties within as little as 30 minutes of being introduced to the body; then you will find out what your body is made of.

As I have said our body eliminates toxins first from the primary chimneys: intestinal tract, urinary tract. When those don't work then the secondary chimneys kick in: respiratory system, skin. The function of healing your body naturally is to:

Avoid toxic exposure

Support defensive body functions

Support elimination functions

So when you see the issues with your lungs, your endurance, and your skin; this is a sign that you're not functioning at the optimal levels.

You can be sure your primary chimneys are functioning by watching for the proper flow of the intestinal tract, proper flow of urine and proper liver function. Skin eruptions are always a sign your body is not aligned. Think about when you were a teenager. Your hormones were all over the place. You rarely think back to those days, but it is all about this primary system, and your endocrine system.

I am sure you rarely think about the endocrine system. Imagine walking down the street in your town yelling at friends, "Hey, how's your endocrine system?" But this system influences almost every cell, organ, and function of our bodies. The endocrine system is instrumental in regulating mood, growth and development, tissue function, metabolism, and sexual function and reproductive processes. When a teenager's body is overflowing with these excess hormones, their livers should quickly react and remove the excess hormones from their body, but they can't. What was your diet like as a teen? How many toxins were in your body at that age? The more toxic, the less ability to detoxify, the more those androgens are going to be going out of that secondary chimney, your skin.

We're craving this feeling of health, and some of us have never had it.

Food as a Digestive Enzyme Complex is amazingness!! A happy GI + Natural Enzyme = ❤

A natural enzyme complex has several different digestive enzymes that work for a variety of items. Normally we are born with these enzymes and they should function properly until we are in our 70's or 80's. Without these enzymes you would have to eat an 80% raw diet to get these enzymes into your body, which isn't practical for most of us. The other option is to supplement with food complexes in capsule and chewable form. Mine contain enzymes including bromelain, papain, lipase, amylase, protease and cellulase. Enzymes are a support substance for the flavonoids in our food. They are sometimes referred to as Vitamin P, but it's not really a vitamin but yet something else that our body requires but cannot produce. So we must eat bioflavonoids or supplement with flavonoid rich whole foods supplements. Enzymes are proteins, and they function within a narrow pH and temperature range as well which is why they function better when we focus on eating mostly plants.

Many enzymes are produced in the digestive system of infants and some, mostly European, adult humans. Enzymes are essential to the complete digestion of whole milk, although what we know now is that there is probably a reason why it's only in most infant's systems. We were not really built, speaking in a Paleolithic manner, to digest milk. If you know much about milk then you have heard the term lactose or lactase before. Lactase is the enzyme found on the walls of our intestines that breaks down the lactose sugar found in milk into galactose and glucose. Despite what you have been told, glucose is NOT the preferred fuel of human metabolism, fat is. Our activity of lactase becomes reduced after we stop breastfeeding, because at that point the body no longer needs as much lactase. This is a genetically programmed event and so it's perfectly natural that 75 % of the Earth's population is lactose intolerant. This is exactly why I want you to just dump the dairy at least while you are trying to figure out what is going on with your body.

As well, calcium can build up in your pineal gland, which is deeply connected to your third eye. If you are trying to activate your inner knowing, decalcifying your pineal gland is on your agenda. Your pineal gland also is responsible for synthesizing melatonin. This gland has the highest calcification rate among all of our organs and tissues, and pineal calcification jeopardizes melatonin's synthetic capacity and is associated with a variety of neuronal diseases. So rise up your awareness, and help your body get to bed and enjoy the recovery that it needs by ditching the dairy for this program. Win-win.

A whole food is just what it sounds like – a food that you eat whole, just the way nature intended. When foods are processed they are often stripped of nutrients and filled with additives, and so you want to eat things that are as close to their natural state as possible. Fruits and vegetables are perfect examples. You can eat them fresh from the garden, skin and all. Eating a diet rich with fruits, vegetables and loads of fiber will support the release of the sludge in your body while refueling you in the best possible way. The vitamins, minerals and phytonutrients in these foods are not only the best for building muscle, but have been shown to protect the body against a variety of chronic diseases including cancer and heart disease.

There are whole foods and then there is what I like to call "Fat-Blocker Foods". These foods fill you up and block absorption of some of those starches and fats. They will give you the easiest way you'll ever find to shed pound after pound and reach your healthy weight goal. This is all about the fiber. Don't jump into 35 grams of fiber on day one of your new journey, because the likely next state will be constipation. Ease in, drink lots of hydrating liquids, and you will pull the sludge out of your colon while feeding the good bacteria in your digestive and elimination tract. As well, fiber reduces your net carbs if you are leaning into the ketogenic version of plant heavy.

You can do this not by eating less but actually by eating more of certain foods. Researchers have found dozens of great tasting foods with an amazing combination of benefits. They are delicious and also block the absorption of fat and calories in the other foods you eat. And these same foods leave you feeling full and totally satisfied for much longer so you eat less. It's a win-win situation.

Certain foods that are high in fiber can "block fat" by helping control your fat and sugar intake. According to the Harvard School of Public Health, women should eat at least 20 grams of fiber per day and men should eat at least 30 grams of fiber each day. Fruits and vegetables are among the healthiest and best fat blocking foods on Earth and are loaded with fiber. Some of these that are highest in fiber are going to contain the most fat blocking abilities are the ones I love the most. Those include:

Raspberries, which have 8 grams of fiber per 1 cup serving
Pears, which have 6 grams of fiber
Apples, which have 5 grams of fiber
Strawberries, with 4 grams of fiber per 1 cup serving
Artichokes, with 10 grams of fiber per serving
Peas, with 9 grams of fiber per 1 cup serving
Broccoli, with 5 grams of fiber per 1 cup serving.

12

Final Countdown

Once you are eating well, you can ease into movement and start working on living your best life. There really are only two major killers in our society: disease and frailty. One or the other is going to most likely take you. If you learn to take care of your emotional self, let love be the guide to where you go, and eat well; then all that is left is movement/breathing.

Frailty is a vitally important issue in the treatment of the elderly. It is something that most people who live to an advanced age will probably face. Frailty can strongly affect how an elderly person will respond to medical treatment, as well as how long and how well they will live. Surprisingly, though common, it remains poorly understood.

Part of the problem is that it defies exact definition. Frailty is not really a disease but rather a combination of the natural aging process and a variety of medical problems. Frailty may not be a disease, but there is no question that certain diseases and medical problems play a large role in it. When you cannot move in the manner you desire, your happiness and all of those brilliant vibrations will decrease.

A common characteristic of muscle from sedentary elderly subjects is a phenomenon called fiber type grouping. Muscles of young and middle-aged subjects contain a mix of fibers types, and therefore have a checkerboard appearance. In untrained elderly subjects clumps of muscle fibers have been observed and consist of predominantly slow twitch or type I fibers. This type of muscle fiber distribution has also been shown in patients with certain neural diseases. Did you forget that I am also a Certified Personal Trainer? So of course we are going into movement.

So what is the solution? It has been shown that resistance training can enhance muscle mass and function even in 90 year old subjects, and is the most effective way to maintain the quality of life as we age.

Research has shown that strengthening exercises are both safe and effective for women and men of all ages, including those who are not in perfect health. In fact, people with health concerns—including heart disease or arthritis—often benefit the most from an exercise program that includes lifting weights a few times each week. And that's not just picking up the remote. Recent studies have even shown that those with chronic fatigue and fibromyalgia can get some relief from strength training. The secret is in minimizing the eccentric muscle loading. You can do this by limiting overhead arm work and exercises done with limbs farther away from the body's midline. Big tip is that you should not attempt to do strength training during a symptom flare.

For most of us strength training, particularly in conjunction with regular gentle aerobic exercise, can also have a profound impact on a person's mental and emotional health.

There are numerous benefits to strength training regularly, particularly as you grow older. It can be very powerful in reducing the signs and symptoms of numerous diseases and chronic conditions, resulting in significant disability and, in some cases, fatal complications. Strengthening exercises, when done properly and through the full range of motion, increases a person's flexibility and balance, which decrease the likelihood and severity of falls. One study in New Zealand worked with a group and they found that the items that strength training can help with are:

Arthritis

Diabetes

Osteoporosis

Obesity

Back pain

Depression

Could you use a little help to eliminate any of those factors?

Beyond the "happy factor" of being connected to health through your fitness we have found that by doing strength and balance training you can reduce your risk of other injuries. You see, as people age, poor balance and flexibility contribute to falls and broken bones. These fractures are common and can lead to a quick downhill slide. Yet one study in New Zealand in women of women 80 years of age and older showed a 40% reduction in falls with simple strength and balance training.

Also, let's talk about what happens to women as we age... we start to widen. I know you don't want to talk about that, but don't we? We need strength training to keep our metabolism burning. Your fat cells are going to do everything in their power to take control of the lower hormone situation. Your muscles job is to boost the metabolism and keep that calorie burning fire stocked. So the type of strength training I recommend you to go for involved in isolating and targeting specific muscle groups using weights like barbells or dumbbells for resistance. You can also use resistance bands which are easy to pack and go with you anywhere.

Strength training for woman is one you wouldn't want to do without, contrary to what the myth says - that it would give you big bulky muscles! You do not have enough testosterone to build up that kind of bulk without supplementing. This type of training will not only help you to ignite your metabolism, and define and tighten your muscles, it also improves your posture and balance and strengthens your bones to better combat the assault of osteoporosis , as you get older. Did you hear that? Improves your posture and balance? It also strengthens your bones. I always include strength training in my toning routine, specifically for exercises that involve the chest, shoulders, arms and upper back. If you are serious about changing your body composition, and how you'll look and feel in the future, then there's no question about it.

The next thing I want to touch base on is having a fit heart, fit lungs and endurance. I will tell you that the best part of my cardio workout is the feeling I get from it. I love endorphins. Hey, I confess. If you have to be addicted to something, why not something good for you, right?

Endorphins are the body's natural pain medication hormones. Endorphins, when they're released, make us feel better, improve our mood, increase pleasure, and minimize pain. There are some good ways, and bad ways, to increase endorphins. And let me tell you a secret, those low endorphin levels make us crave unhealthy fat.

High concentrations of endorphins in the brain produce a sense of euphoria, enhance pleasure, and suppress pain, both emotionally and physically. When endorphins are low, people feel anxious; they are also more aware of pain. They have an appetite for fat and fatty foods, such as fries, cheese, creamy sauces, margarine, butter, fried chicken, potato chips, and chocolate, to name some of the most popular examples. Upon eating some fat, they will notice a change in mood, feeling more pleasure. This feeling is related to a higher concentration of endorphins. Exercise, by releasing fat from within the body, raises endorphins and causes the same mood changes. There are more reasons besides the calorie burn to get your workout in. And the foods that we eat are produced to make you feel that way, and so if you can find a way to feel better when you have cravings for potato chips and chocolate, then wouldn't you want to give it a try?

IF YOU WALK, RUN, DANCE, PLAY TENNIS, HIKE, BIKE, OR SWIM, then the health experts say you are moving toward living longer and in better health. A program of regular aerobic exercise can help you avoid chronic diseases, such as heart disease, hypertension, stroke, diabetes, and some cancers. Aerobic exercise can also lower blood pressure, build stronger bones, improve muscle strength and flexibility, lessen depression, and help control your weight. When I started dancing this year, about ten months ago; my body would start playing the music in my head when it wanted more. You have to learn to be aware and tune into your body, and its needs.

Aerobic exercise involves continuous, rhythmic activity of large muscles in the legs and buttocks to strengthen your heart and lungs (cardiovascular system). When you exercise, the muscles demand more oxygen-rich blood and give off more carbon dioxide and other waste. This makes your heartbeat faster to keep up with the blood circulation. This is totally better than coffee in my opinion, and easier on your adrenals when done properly.

When you follow a program of regular aerobic exercise, over time your heart grows stronger and can meet the muscles' demands without as much effort. Both men and women can benefit from cardiovascular fitness.

Safe and effective aerobic training guidelines include frequency, intensity, and time (FIT):

Frequency: Exercise at least three times a week.

Intensity: Exercise hard enough to reach your target heart rate. Cardio fat burning ranges are not as high as you think.

Time: Include at least 20 minutes of aerobic exercise in each session.

Aerobic exercise refers to the initial phase of exercise, or to any short burst of intense exertion, in which the glycogen or sugar is used without oxygen, and is a far less efficient process. Higher intensity exercise, such as High-intensity interval training (HIIT), increases the resting metabolic rate (RMR) in the 24 hours following high intensity exercise, ultimately burning more calories than lower intensity aerobic exercise; low intensity exercise burns more calories during the exercise, due to the increased duration, but fewer afterwards. So HIIT is the kind of workout that is going to improve your athletic endurance as well as your fat-burning potential. But like a hard strength training workout, which will also keep your metabolism increased over the next day. Working out for twenty minutes allows your body's gatekeepers to open the storage cells and release what they've stored in your cells. So this time frame is essential to build up to, even if it is just walking.

Apart from the fat-burn issue, endurance aerobics and extensive cardio workouts may condition your body for distance, but they do not help with lung capacity. Your heart and lungs were designed for short bursts of intense exercise followed by rest. Another reason I love HIIT. Burst, rest, burst rest. This resting period is critical for the body's ability to strengthen lung capacity, quite the opposite of what many endurance athletes achieve. If your body isn't pushed hard enough to be gasping, the lungs never expand fully to reach reserve capacity.

There have been multiple studies comparing the traditional endurance training versus high intensity interval training. Some years ago, Harvard researchers published a study involving over 7,000 participants. The conclusion of the study found that preventing heart disease is based on the level of intensity, not endurance aerobic activity.

A study at McMaster University in 2006 demonstrated that just 2.5 hours of sprint interval training can yield similar biochemical muscle changes to 10.5 hours of endurance training and similar endurance performance benefits. Do you want to workout for 2.5 hours or 10.5 hours?

I generally connect my HIIT days to my lessened days of core work, and strength training, usually leg day. If I do short strength training I'll add in a little jumping around. If I am looking for aerobics I will dance. Dancing is so gentle on my adrenals, and I love the music.

Stretching can also be hard for a lot of us. You have to do this since it's the only way you get the lubrication your joints need. And it's only after you lose that use of a joint that you realize how important it is. Flexibility is defined as the range of motion available around a joint. Good flexibility and muscle length ensure proper joint lubrication and health, and optimal muscle contractile function lubricating the joints. You have to be flexible to be able to keep your balance which requires a combination of a strong core, and the ability to reach. Having flexibility lowers your risk of falling. And with these moments of clarity that you get when you are slowing down, lengthening your muscles by stopping and breathing (even if you are moving as moving mediation is what I like to call stretching).

Breathing is just as essential as the movement. If you start there, you are already ahead of the game. Breathing will balance your autonomic nervous system, and it is actually how your body removes the sludge outside of the waste/fiber factor. Remember that the recent results, published in the British Medical Journal, reveal that 22 pounds (10 kg) of fat turns into 18.5 pounds (8.4 kg) of carbon dioxide, which is exhaled when we breathe, and 3.5 pounds (1.6 kg) of water, which we then excrete through our urine, tears, sweat and other bodily fluids. If all of life is as simple as remembering to stop and breathe to return our machine bodies back to happiness, then the rest will follow.

As they say, "Inhale the future, exhale the past." The rest will be created.

References

1 - Copper Stress Induces a Global Stress Response in Staphylococcus aureus and Represses sae and agr Expression and Biofilm Formation. Department of Genetics, University of Leicester, University Road, Leicester LE1 7RH, United Kingdom,1 Department of Biological Sciences, Illinois State University, Normal, Illinois 617902

2 - PRASAD R , SINGH A, DAS B K, UPADHYAY R S,SINGH T B , MISHRA O P. CEREBROSPINAL FLUID AND SERUM ZINC, COPPER, MAGNESIUM AND CALCIUM LEVELS IN CHILDREN WITH IDIOPATHIC SEIZURE. Journal of Clinical and Diagnostic Research [serial online] 2009 December [cited: 2017 Nov 29]; 3:1841-1846.

3 - Systemic Staphylococcus aureus infection mediated by Candida albicans hyphal invasion of mucosal tissue Microbiology. 2015 Jan; 161(Pt 1): 168–181. doi: 10.1099/mic.0.083485-0

4 - Selenium Deficiency and Toxicity in the Environment Fiona Fordyce, British Geological Survey

5 - Association between thyroid function and gallstone disease, Henry Völzke, Daniel M Robinson, and Ulrich John; World J Gastroenterol. 2005 Sep 21; 11(35): 5530–5534.

6 - The neuroprotective effects of cocoa flavanol and its influence on cognitive performance, Astrid Nehlig; Br J Clin Pharmacol. 2013 Mar; 75(3): 716–727.

7 - A new mechanism for diverticular diseases: aging-related vagal withdrawal. Yun AJ1, Bazar KA, Lee PY. Med Hypotheses. 2005;64(2):252-5.

8 - Tony Valente, Juan Hidalgo, Irene Bolea, Bartolomé Ramirez, Neus Anglés, Jordi Reguant, José Ramón Morelló, Cristina Gutiérrez, Mercè Boada and Mercedes Unzeta. A Diet Enriched in Polyphenols and Polyunsaturated Fatty Acids, LMN Diet, Induces Neurogenesis in the Subventricular Zone and Hippocampus of Adult Mouse Brain. Journal of Alzheimer's Disease, 2009; 18 (4) DOI: 10.3233/JAD-2009-1188

9 - The neurobiological link between compassion and love, Tobias Esch and George B. Stefano; Med Sci Monit. 2011; 17(3): RA65–RA75.

10 - Polyphenols and Sunburn, Suzana Saric and Raja K. Sivamani; Int J Mol Sci. 2016 Sep; 17(9): 1521.

11 - Flavonoid intake and ovarian cancer risk in a population-based case-control study
Margaret A. Gates Allison F. Vitonis, Shelley S. Tworoger, Bernard Rosner, Linda Titus-Ernstoff, Susan E. Hankinson, and

Daniel W. Cramer; Int J Cancer. Author manuscript; available in PMC 2010 Apr 15.

12 - Apigenin inhibits the self-renewal capacity of human ovarian cancer SKOV3-derived sphere-forming cells. Tang AQ, Cao XC, Tian L, He L, Liu F.; Mol Med Rep. 2015 Mar;11(3):2221-6. doi: 10.3892/mmr.2014.2974. Epub 2014 Nov 18.

13 - The interface between the immune system and autonomic nervous system. Nakane S, Mukaino A, Ando Y; Nihon Rinsho Meneki Gakkai Kaishi. 2017;40(5):352-360. doi: 10.2177/jsci.40.352.

14 - Altered glutathione homeostasis in animals prenatally exposed to lipopolysaccharide. Zhu Y, Carvey PM, Ling Z. Neurochem Int. 2007 Mar;50(4):671-80. Epub 2007 Jan 13.

15 - Autoimmunity and the Gut Andrew W. Campbell. Autoimmune Dis. 2014; 2014: 152428.

16 - The Potential Roles of Bisphenol A (BPA) Pathogenesis in Autoimmunity, Datis Kharrazian. Autoimmune Diseases

Volume 2014 (2014), Article ID 743616

17 - Epstein-Barr Virus Infection is Common in Inflamed Gastrointestinal Mucosa. Julie L. Ryan, PhD, MPH, You-Jun Shen, MD, Douglas R. Morgan, MD, MPH, Leigh B. Thorne, MD, Shannon C. Kenney, MD, Ricardo L. Dominguez, MD, and Margaret L. Gulley, MD; Dig Dis Sci. Author manuscript; available in PMC 2013 Jul 1.

18 - The association of asthma, total IgE, and blood lead and cadmium levels. Warren Alpert Medical School of Brown University, Providence, RI; www.jacionline.org/article/S0091-6749(16)30421-3/pdf by S Park

19 - The role of vitamin D on circulating memory T cells in children: The Generation R study.

Looman KIM1, Jansen MAE, Voortman T, van den Heuvel D, Jaddoe VWV,, Franco OH,, van Zelm MC, Moll HA.Pediatr Allergy Immunol. 2017 Sep;28(6):579-587. doi: 10.1111/pai.12754. Epub 2017 Aug 7.

20 - Homocysteine levels are associated with MTHFR A1298C polymorphism in Indian population. Jitender Kumar Æ Swapan K. Das,Priyanka Sharma, Ganesan Karthikeyan, Lakshmy Ramakrishnan, Shantanu Sengupta. J Hum Genet (2005) 50:655–663

21 - Frequent consumption of milk, yogurt, cold breakfast cereals, peppers, and cruciferous vegetables and intakes of dietary folate and riboflavin but not vitamins B-12 and B-6 are inversely associated with serum total homocysteine concentrations in the US population. Ganji V, Kafai MR. Am J Clin Nutr. 2004 Dec;80(6):1500-7.

22 - Asparagine bioavailability governs metastasis in a model of breast cancer. Simon R. V. Knott, Elvin Wagenblast, Showkhin Khan, Sun Y. Kim, Mar Soto, Michel Wagner, Marc-Olivier Turgeon, Lisa Fish, Nicolas Erard, Annika L. Gable, Ashley R. Maceli, Steffen Dickopf, Evangelia K. Papachristou, Clive S. D'Santos, Lisa A. Carey, John E. Wilkinson, J. Chuck

Harrell, Charles M. Perou, Hani Goodarzi, George
Poulogiannis & Gregory J. Hannon. Nature volume 554,
pages 378–381 (15 February 2018)

23 - Curcumin prevents toxic effects of 2,3,7,8-
tetrachlorodibenzo-p-dioxin (TCDD) on humoral immunity in
rats. Osman Çiftçi

Pages 31-38 | Received 28 May 2010, Published online: 03
Mar 2011

24 - The use of high-selenium yeast to raise selenium
status: how does it measure up? Margaret P. Rayman (a1)
https://doi.org/10.1079/BJN20041251Published online: 01
March 2007

25 - Association of MTHFR gene C677T mutation with
diabetic peripheral neuropathy and diabetic retinopathy

Serbulent Yigit,1 Nevin Karakusand Ahmet Inanir. Mol Vis.
2013; 19: 1626–1630. Published online 2013 Jul 25.

26 - Toxicity of formulants and heavy metals in
glyphosate-based herbicides and other pesticides.
N.DefargeaJ.Spiroux de VendômoisbG.E.Séralinia.
https://doi.org/10.1016/j.toxrep.2017.12.025

27 - Chromium Toxicity. What Are the Physiologic Effects
of Chromium Exposure?
http://web.archive.org/web/20150421022403/http://www.atsdr
.cdc.gov/csem/csem.asp?csem=10&po=10

28 - Augmenting antidepressants with triiodothyronine: An
underutilized strategy

Current Psychiatry. 2011 July;10(7):43-44; by Daniel Gih, MD

29 - The long-term effect of eicosapentaenoic acid on serum levels of lipoprotein (a) and lipids in patients with vascular disease Source: J Atheroscler Thromb. 1996;2(2):107-9.

Shinozaki K1, Kambayashi J, Kawasaki T, Uemura Y, Sakon M, Shiba E, Shibuya T, Nakamura T, Mori T

Abstra

ABOUT THE AUTHOR

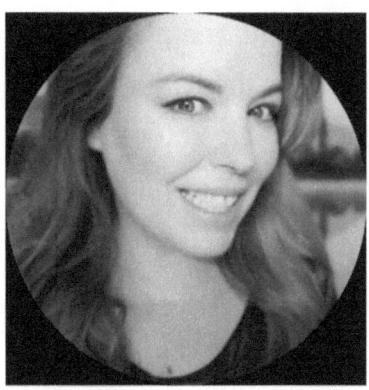

Barbara Christensen is an Energetic and Holistic Facilitator who specializes in the energy body connection. She struggled with her health throughout her childhood and early adulthood which lead her to seek out and become a purpose driven alternative expert. Barbara has been trained in the areas of nutrition, aromatherapy, energy modalities and anatomy; and specializes in whole body wellness. She says, "My belief is that most of what we are dealing with is passed down and environmental gene expression that can be changed with diet, mindset and alternative therapies." Her expertise has made her a sought after guide for vegan paleo dieters, and those seeking to awaken and create a higher energy vibration.

Barbara homeschools her daughter with special learning and allergy needs, having watched too many kids go through the public system without the personalized support they need. It was the same spark that sparked her creation of the Paleo Vegeo dietary lifestyle and the plant-heavy Ketolicious Reset program. Barbara runs the largest vegan paleo challenge group on Facebook, where you can get support in finding your own path forward. Learn more: www.PaleoVegeo.com

Barbara has found a life balance that allows her to work with clients from all over the world via the internet and online conferencing, for aromatherapy, wellness work and with distance energy models. She specializes in seeking the answers through her claircognizance abilities for mastering wellness readings. Learn more: www.BijaCoaching.com.

www.ingramcontent.com/pod-product-compliance
Lightning Source LLC
Chambersburg PA
CBHW021404210526
45463CB00001B/219